BEYOND AMALGAM

By Susan Stockton, MA

D1636820

Beyond Amalgam
by
Susan Stockton

Copyright© 1998 by Susan Stockton

All Rights Reserved
Printed in the United Sates of America
Revised Edition - 2000
Third Printing - 2001

No part of this book may be reproduced stored in retrieval system, or transmitted, in any form or by any means, either electronic, mechanical, photocopying, micro-filming, recording, or otherwise, without written permission from the publisher.

ISBN 0-9628770-2-6

Library of Congress Catalog Card Number: 00-102935

Beyond Amalgam is not intended as medical advice. It is written solely for informational and educational purposes. Please consult a health professional should the need for one be indicated.

Power of One Publishing
c/o Renew Life
2076 Sunnydale Drive
Clearwater, FL 33765-1204
1-800-830-4778
susan@healthcarealternatives.net

Dedication

This book is dedicated to those pioneers in non-toxic dentistry who have had the vision to see what IS - despite being taught it ISN'T - and the courage to do something about it!

Acknowledgement

Many thanks to Judy Koster, RN, and to Ruth Swimmer for their help with proofing this manuscript. I am grateful, too, to the many readers who have provided feedback and input for this book.

I am indebted, too, to Kenn and Vi Rust of Rust Graphics in Denver, CO for getting this and my other manuscripts ready for the printer.

A huge "thank you" goes also to my dear friend and former publisher, Sandy Knowles, for working overtime to get this book and others in print. I must acknowledge her also for the fine work she's done in designing and executing my website. Her skill and generosity have kept my work alive!

I must also acknowledge John Augspurger, DDS, of Colorado Springs, CO for the outstanding prosthetic work he has provided. He is truly a master craftsman.

And finally, my undying gratitude to Dr. Wes Shankland, who very likely saved my life, for his loving care and help with this manuscript.

TABLE OF CONTENTS

*"Beware of bargains in fire extinguishers,
life preservers, brain operations,
parachutes and dental care."*

The Holistic Dental Digest Plus, May-June, 2000

PREFACE

Our mechanistic view of life has given rise to the concept of the human body as a series of connecting, but independent parts. In line with this fragmented, compartmentalized view of the body, we have created specialists who deal exclusively with the various parts of it. The teeth, gums and jaw are generally considered the domain of dentists with various specialties, while other body parts fall under the jurisdiction of a myriad of specialties within the medical field. In keeping with this traditional paradigm, MDs will generally not question their patients about dental problems, nor will dentists ask their patients about their systemic problems (except to rule out certain heart conditions which alert them to the "need" to use antibiotics before and after treatment).

The concept that patients' health problems could be caused by hidden dental problems is certainly not compatible with this paradigm and therefore is generally dismissed out of hand by most dentists and doctors – even so-called "holistic" ones. Nevertheless, there is overwhelming evidence that a great many of today's health problems have their origin in the mouth, stemming from the effects of toxic dental materials and/or the disease conditions resulting from the standard practices of root canal fillings and tooth extractions. The focus of this book is on extractions as they are commonly performed and the cavitations, holes in the jawbone that do not completely heal over with new bone, which result. Although hidden (usually not apparent on x-ray, nor causing local symptoms), there are indications that cavitations from old extractions are a serious and widespread problem. Because of their obscurity and practitioners' lack of familiarity with them, these holes in the jawbone routinely elude detection. The patient is thus often misdiagnosed and therefore mistreated – or even told it's "all in his head."

People whose health conditions are caused by cavitations are most likely those who have failed to respond to conventional – and even alternative – treatment modalities: The *effect* will not be eliminated until the *cause* is identified and removed. This will not happen to any great degree until a significant paradigm shift occurs, until fragmentation yields to 'holism,' until dentists begin questioning their patients about their systemic problems, and doctors start questioning theirs about their dental problems.

"Eighty percent of patient illness I find in my practice originates in the mouth. Daily I continue to be astounded at the world wide impairment that oral disease has on human health."

— Dr. Christopher Hussar

FOREWORD

by Christopher John Hussar, DDS, DO

Deep within the jawbones of many of us — and below the level of our awareness — lurk insidious lesions that slowly erode, creating holes which cause local tissue destruction and lead to systemic toxicity.

The formation of these lesions frequently begins with extraction of "wisdom" teeth (which may be more aptly referred to as "teeth of misfortune," in consideration of the problems so frequently resulting from their removal). Although these teeth are generally extracted either due to eruption or because they are impacted into the jawbone, the oral surgeon often fails to recognize them as a source of infection. Biopsy of the bone surrounding an erupted or impacted wisdom tooth will, however, usually reveal presence of disease. Such disease may range in manifestation from a dying tooth with chronic pulpitis (inflamed pulp) to one surrounded by full blown necrotic (dying), ischemic (lacking oxygen) bone. Although these teeth are routinely extracted, the infected bone is left behind, as well as an open hole which serves as an ingress for oral bacteria and an incubation chamber for microbes, leading to further infection, both locally and systemically, and eventually leading to the formation of a "cavitation."

I will never forget the experience of removing a small fragment of a pea and a carrot from a cavitational area. Somewhere later in life, a patient such as this one will begin to experience facial pain, or perhaps chronic sinusitis or migraine headaches, or arthritic conditions, or fibromyalgia, or low back pain, or may end up in a wheelchair with signs and symptoms of multiple sclerosis or amyotrophic lateral sclerosis (a.k.a. ALS or Lou Gehrig's disease). These patients run the gamut from doctor to doctor, from specialist to specialist, collecting a myriad of diagnoses, without anyone having a clue as to what treatment is really appropriate. Consequently, the patient goes on a search for the "Grail" or solution to health problems, which may lead to years and years of drugs and hundreds of thousands of dollars spent without a successful outcome, with no satisfactory answer to the question, "Why am I sick?" Some fortunate few may end up in the hands of a dental surgeon who specializes in performing surgery on the jaw, removing these lesions known as dental cavitations.

Over the years of performing such jawbone surgery, I have been privileged to be able to remove small areas of chronically infected dead bone from people's jaws, resulting in the cure of such diverse conditions as head-aches, blindness, migratory arthritis, autoimmune disease, tinnitus, fibromyalgia, ear pain, neck pain and many others. I have performed oral surgery on patients and have subsequently seen what appeared to be a cancerous mass essentially disappear from that patient's abdomen.

Painful facial conditions are widespread, as evidenced by the many pages of Internet entries of such patients. Most of these people can either be cured or substantially improved by a simple oral surgical procedure done within the confines of the jawbone. This usually entails going into the jaw, gaining access to the interior aspect of the jawbone with a small window and cleaning out dead, chronically disease-infected bone.

The existence of these jawbone lesions has been known to the medical and dental profession for centuries and is reflected in articles written by both physicians and dentists alike throughout history. Such articles not only recognize the existence of these lesions, but their systemic effects as well. Nonetheless, the powers-that-be of the American Dental Association persist in denying the existence of cavitations. The unfortunate result is that people suffering with chronic infections in their jawbones are told by their dentist or oral surgeon there is "nothing wrong" with their jaw or with their root canal based upon the (mis)interpretation of a dental x-ray.

Beyond Amalgam is very informative and presents the subject of jawbone cavitations succinctly for all to understand, from the experienced to the novitiate. The quality of writing should appeal to clinician, patient and interested reader alike.

This book is written from the author's viewpoint, based upon her experiences with jawbone cavitations and their disastrous effects upon her health. Reading about these experiences elicits empathy for her and for all of us who have suffered from this debilitating disease. This book will serve to bring to light an insidious hidden pathology that affects millions of Americans and people throughout the world.

Susan Stockton is to be lauded for her perseverance in seeking out her health "Grail," if you will, realizing that cavitations were the substantial part of her answer to achieving wellness. By writing this book, Susan will give hope to others suffering from the myriad of symptoms typically displayed by those afflicted with this disease. Hopefully, these patients will eventually end up in the trained hands of a cavitational surgeon and be cured.

I first encountered the word "cavitation" several years ago when I read Dr. Hulda Clark's book, *The Cure for All Cancers*, written in 1993. This then unknown author, a naturopathic physician with a doctorate in physiology, would later write three more books, *The Cure for All Diseases, The Cure for HIV/AIDS* and *The Cure for All Advanced Cancers,* all of which would quickly become bestsellers, making her a prominent (albeit controversial) figure in the alternative health field.

A COMMON THEME

All of Dr. Clark's books share a common theme: Disease is caused largely by parasites. Taken at face value, this hypothesis would lead to the conclusion that the way to cure disease is to simply kill parasites. It is important to understand, however, that parasite treatment by itself is insufficient to eradicate disease *conditions.* And Dr. Clark is well aware of this. She states quite plainly in her writings that the proliferation of parasites is caused by the presence of solvents, such as propyl alcohol, in body tissues. And she gives the reader much detailed information about how to avoid exposure to these solvents. Despite this fact, many of her readers are only "getting" the part about parasites and are failing to abandon use of solvent-containing products. Even among those who *are* being conscientious, there are many who are not getting yet another important part of Dr. Clark's message: Parasites cannot be eliminated from the body until cavitations are eliminated.

LACK OF INFORMATION

I am convinced that many avid Dr. Clark fans are failing to take this important step due to an inadequate understanding of the role cavitations play in creating and perpetuating health problems, as well as the fact that there exists in this country a dearth of qualified dental practitioners to adequately treat the problem.

And then there is the rest of the population, those who have never read Dr. Clark's books and have never heard the word "cavitation." To them this is completely uncharted territory. I therefore offer this book as a roadmap which will hopefully guide readers to an understanding of the nature and effects of cavitations, arm them with information about how to identify and possibly correct the condition, and most important of all, prevent its recurrence.

TOO LITTLE ABOUT CAVITATIONS

Hulda Clark defines cavitations as "holes left in the jawbone by an incompletely extracted tooth,"[1] citing one of the technical terms for the condition, "alveolar cavitational osteopathosis." She goes on to say:

> *A properly cleaned socket which is left after an extraction will heal and fill with bone. Dentists routinely do NOT clean the socket of tissue remnants or infected bone. A dry socket (really an infected socket) is a common result. These sockets never fully heal. Thirty years after an extraction, a cavitation will still be there. It is a form of osteomyelitis, which means bone infection.*

The above information is all that was given about cavitations in the first edition of Dr. Clark's 510-page book, *The Cure for All Cancers*. This little bit of vitally important and incomplete information easily gets lost and obscured amid the volumes of other important data in this book and in her others. I have discovered, however, that Dr. Clark's most recent edition of *The Cure for All Cancers*, introduced in early 1998, includes an expanded dental section with additional information on cavitations, as does her latest book, *The Cure for All Advanced Cancers*.

Ironically, at the time I first read Dr. Clark's words about cavitations I was unknowingly suffering from the systemic effects of advanced severe "alveolar cavitational osteopathosis" (more simply referred to as 'osteitis' or cavitations). Even when I became aware of the problem, finding a dentist who could appropriately treat the condition proved problematic.

I finally found such a dentist in mid 1997. After surgical treatment of eleven cavitations and years of suffering, the desperate search for the cause of my health problems came to an end – and the work of repairing years of damage began. The dentist who treated me is one of a handful of modern-day pioneers in the surgical treatment of cavitations. In the ten years he has been treating the condition, many grateful patients with a variety of ailments have credited him with their recovery.

NOT A NEW CONDITION

The original pioneers in cavitation research are no longer living. As with much other critically important information in the fields of medicine and dentistry, information on cavitations has been around for a long time – but buried (like the information on the dangers of mercury-containing "silver" amalgam fillings).

Although the public's *awareness* of the dangers posed by the mercury in amalgams *began* with Dr. Hal Huggins's book, *It's All in Your Head,* the dangers of mercury have actually been *long* known to medicine. This heavy metal was identified as a *neurotoxicant* (poison to the nervous system) in the 17th century when 'hatters' in France were becoming "mad" from inhaling the fumes of the mercury compound used in preparation of felt hats.

Like Clark, Huggins mentions cavitations in his book(2), but gives insufficient information to alert the reader to the magnitude of the problem. In his discussion of the subject, he states that he found both Amyotrophic Lateral Sclerosis (ALS or Lou Gehrig's Disease) and Parkinson's Disease to be unresponsive to mercury removal alone; both, however, responded well when cavitations were surgically treated as well. He describes the surgical treatment as a "simple five-minute procedure" wherein the *periodontal ligament* (attaching the tooth to the jawbone) is removed. This ligament is like a hammock in which the tooth sits. Once the tooth is removed, it no longer serves a purpose and, if left in, will most likely cause problems sooner or later. Huggins compares this membrane to the afterbirth that follows the delivery of a baby, explaining that if this afterbirth is left in, death of the mother will probably ensue. Leaving the periodontal ligament in, while not fatal, does form a barrier to new bone growth, so that incomplete healing of the socket occurs. What happens is that the top of the socket tends to "seal over two or three millimeters of bone; under that, a hole remains."(3)   Inside these holes or cavitations, adverse cellular changes occur, and infection often develops due to severe restriction of blood flow to the area. The site then becomes a focal point of low grade infection which can affect the entire body.

Dr. Huggins has apparently delved more deeply into the subject of cavitations since publication of *It's All in Your Head*. A very informative video on the subject, featuring Thomas Levy, MD in a 4/97 dental seminar, is available through Huggins' Institute. The toll-free order number is 1-800-331-2303.

In the same year Huggins' book came out (1993), another was introduced that would awaken the public to an equally dangerous practice of modern dentistry: root canals.

BURIED TOOTH TRUTH

Endodontist (root canal specialist) George E. Meinig, wrote *Root Canal Cover Up* after reviewing 25 years of neglected root canal research conducted by the late Dr. Weston Price, former Director of Research for the American Dental Association. Price's research spanned a time frame from the 1920s to the 40s. It established a link between root canal-filled teeth and heart, kidney and uterine disease, as well as disorders of the nervous and endocrine systems. He found that root canal-filled teeth *always* remain infected and organ damage results from migration of toxins from these teeth to distant organs. Price, author of 220 scientific articles (and the 526-page classic treatise on nutrition, *Nutrition and Physical Degeneration*), did his root canal research in conjunction with sixty of the country's top scientists under the auspices of the American Dental Association and its Research Institute. In addition, "His research was extensively documented in two volumes, totaling 1174 pages and in 25 scientific articles appearing in dental and medical literature."(4)

Despite all of this, Price's root canal research was buried, forced underground 70 years ago, because the central thesis of the work – the *focal infection* theory – was incompatible with dominant medical theory and teachings of the time. According to Meinig, who is one of the 19 founding members of the American Association of Endodontists, the Root Canal Association is *still* covering up the relevance of Price's work and denying its validity. They have *not*, however, been able to disprove his thesis. Because of the suppression of Price's work, root canals continue to be routinely performed – 25,000,000 of them in 1996, 30,000,000+ projected for 2000 – and people continue to suffer needlessly.

Bacteria from root canal-filled teeth have been demonstrated to invade bone and tissue adjacent to the tooth's root. This bacterial invasion can trigger the formation of cavitations. Also, ironically, when root canal treatment fails, necessitating loss of the tooth, or when the patient elects extraction to avoid or correct the problems posed by root canals, even more problems may result, since the trauma of the surgery, if done using standard extraction technique, can cause spreading of existing cavitations, as well as creation of new ones.

Dr. Meinig states that he knew little about jawbone cavitations when he wrote the first edition of *Root Canal Cover Up*, but after later obtaining information about them, he included it in his second edition, in the form of a rewritten chapter 24. The focal infection theory is central to an understanding of the systemic effects of cavitations, as well as root canals, and will be explored in the pages that follow.

THE NEED TO KNOW MORE

The bottom line is that the average person needs to know a lot more about the dangers of routine dental procedures than he now knows in order to safeguard his health in today's world. And, he needs to know what the alternatives are to toxic dentistry and where he can find skilled, responsible alternative practitioners. It is the purpose of this book to fill some of these needs to some degree. More detailed information will no doubt follow in the form of future books to be written by progressive dentists and others in the field.

Thanks to the efforts of professionals like Huggins and Meinig who had the courage to speak out and spread the truth about mercury and root canals (Huggins lost his license), there is now a growing awareness about these important issues. More and more dentists are establishing mercury-free practices. Fewer, it seems, are yet ready to abandon lucrative root canal practices. Although taught in school, fewer still are properly cleaning out sockets following extractions. And *even fewer* are opening up healed-over extraction sites to dig out dead bone from old cavitations. And yet this is exactly what must be done on a fairly large scale to make significant progress in reversing the downward spiral of our health. It has been suggested that once our society abandons the practice of performing root canals because of the demonstrated health hazards they pose, endodontists can be retrained to surgically treat cavitations. Since virtually everyone who has ever had a tooth extracted (especially "wisdom" teeth) develops cavitations, there will be plenty of business for these dentists once the public is educated on the subject.

EDUCATION VS. PROPAGANDA

Unfortunately, the powers-that-be work at cross purposes to the public's receipt of such an education. The American Dental Association has repeatedly issued public policy statements that bear no resemblance to the truth, denying the dangers posed by their "time honored" practices. (Amalgam may have been in use for 100 years, but that doesn't make it safe: The incidence of degenerative disease has also escalated dramatically in this country over that period of time.)

We accept the proclamations of this dental organization and others because they have the weight of authority behind them. Instead, we need to look at the facts, learn to think for ourselves, become our own authorities and seek out enlightened, aware practitioners who can help us.

MERCURY-FREE ISN'T NECESSARILY HOLISTIC

My own experience has shown that many so-called "holistic" dentists are simply practitioners who have stopped using mercury for filling teeth. Many remain uninformed about the dangers of other toxic dental materials, root canal and fluoride (another neurotoxin) treatments and standard extraction technique. Most dentists in practice in this country today, sadly, are as unaware of the cavitation problem as the average patient – and his doctor. As Dr. Frank Jerome, DDS, author of *Tooth Truth*, puts it, most of these practitioners are merely "tooth mechanics." As such, they are totally unaware of the systemic effect of the treatments they perform.

The truly holistic dentist is one who understands that the mouth is connected to the rest of the body, that foci of infection in this orifice can and do cause and perpetuate many diverse health problems. As Hulda Clark so eloquently states, "Teeth have the same tissue frequency as some distant organs . . . Bacteria take advantage of this common resonance and invade both organs."(5) We will look more closely at this tooth/body connection in the pages that follow.

CHAPTER ONE

*"The holes left behind by formerly extracted
wisdom teeth can be a source of
immunological challenge, as we've seen
in our practice, for 60 years."*
— **Michael G. LaMarche, DDS**

MANY NAMES

Numerous terms have been used over the years to describe jawbone cavitations. They include:

Ischemic osteonecrosis	Alveolar cavitation pathosis
Chronic osteomyelitis	Trigger point bone cavity
Avascular necrosis	Interference field
Intraosseous ischemia	Invisible osteomyelitis
Ratner's bone cavity	Aseptic osteonecrosis
Alveolar osteopathosis	Chronic osteitis
Robert's bone cavity	

Neuralgia Inducing Cavitational Osteonecrosis (NICO)

Most descriptions of the condition incorporate the words "osteomyelitis" and "osteonecrosis." An understanding of these terms is vital, therefore, to an understanding of the condition. "Osteo" means bone. "Necrosis" is death of living tissue. Osteonecrosis is defined as "the death of a portion of [bone] tissue differentially affected by local injury, as loss of blood supply, corrosion, burning or the local lesion of a disease." The same on-line source defines osteomyelitis: "An infectious disease of bone often of bacterial origin that is marked by local death and separation of tissue." In both conditions we have tissue death, but only in the myelitis is the element of infection present.

THE HISTORICAL PERSPECTIVE

Jerry E. Bouquot, DDS, MSD, a former pathology professor at the University of West Virginia, has been a key cavitation researcher since the early 1990s. He is the recognized expert on cavitation pathology on this continent. In a very informative paper entitled *In Review of NICO (Neuralgia-Inducing Cavitational Osteonecrosis), G.V. Black's Forgotten Disease*, written in 1995, Bouquot recounts the history of the disease, observing that "ischemic osteonecrosis [bone death due to poor blood supply] of the femur [leg bone] in children was independently differentiated from osteomyelitis in *1910*."

Twenty years later it was found to also occur in adults. The investigator who made this discovery, Phemister, concluded that osteonecrosis was an avascular [lack of blood supply] phenomenon *rather than an infection*. It was he who coined the term "cavitation." We now know Phemister was correct — Osteonecrosis is indeed characterized by the presence of ischemia. Cavitations are therefore sometimes referred to as "ischemic osteonecrosis" or "avascular necrosis," indicating bone death is due to impaired circulation.

CONSEQUENCES OF POOR BLOOD SUPPLY

The important thing for us to recognize is that restricted blood flow to the affected tissue is the central factor in formation of jawbone cavitations. It is failure of the surgeon to remove the periodontal ligament at the time of tooth extraction that sets up a barrier to the creation of new blood vessels and consequently to the regrowth of bone. Dr. Hal Huggins explains it rather simply:

> *Bone cells will naturally grow to connect with other bone cells after tooth removal – providing they can communicate with each other. If the periodontal ligament is left in the socket, however, bone cells look out and see the ligament so they do not attempt to "heal" by growing to find other bone cells.*(6)

When blood flow to the socket is inhibited, oxygen and nutrients are unavailable to the tissues, and bone death (necrosis) ensues.

Following extraction, bacteria and their toxins become trapped in the periodontal ligament. These bacteria mutate due to the anaerobic (lack of oxygen) conditions and begin the job of decomposing dead tissue. In time, therefore, the periodontal ligament will be broken down, but areas of necrosis will still remain in the bone and can spread to other portions of the jawbone if proper treatment is not received.

This lack of proper healing is not at all apparent from a visual inspection of the mouth. The top of the socket will ultimately heal over with bone and new gum tissue. However, it is only a superficial healing, for holes (cavitations) frequently remain a couple of millimeters below the bony cap of the socket as a result of avascular conditions.

DEADLY TOXINS

Biopsies of tissue removed from jawbone cavitations have revealed the presence of as many as 20-30 species of bacteria.(7) Also found are white blood cells or lymphocytes whose job it is to fight infection. Huggins states,"Monocytes (large white cells with a single nucleus) have been observed to evolve three additional nuclei, a[n] [abnormal] cellular change prompted by the extreme toxicity of the environment."(8) Although bacteria are usually found at cavitation sites, they are characteristically few in number. More of a problem than the bacteria are the toxins they produce. When aerobic bacteria (those needing oxygen) get trapped in an anaerobic environment (the cavitation site), the result is the production of deadly chemical toxins. These toxins become particularly virulent when they intermingle with heavy metals and other toxins in the mouth.

The preliminary research of Dr. Boyd Haley of the University of Kentucky, who is currently doing a great deal of work on classifying and typing the toxins from bacteria in cavitations (and root canals), shows that these strains are more toxic than botulism . . . "Some of the most toxic substances known to man."(9) These toxins are described as "extremely dangerous," even in very low concentrations. Some are "100 to 1000 times more toxic than botulism in their effects on enzyme systems,"(10) according to Thomas Levy, MD, alluding to unpublished research by Hal Huggins. The systemic effect of these toxins can be quite devastating and will be discussed shortly. Let's return now, however, to the historical perspective on cavitations.

LOST IN TIME

In *1920*, ten years before Phemister coined the term "cavitation" and described the phenomenon as primarily an avascular, rather than an infectious one, another researcher, G.V. Black, had described it as a "cell by cell bone death." This "chronic osteitis," as he called it, differed from osteomyelitis in its "unique ability to produce extensive bone destruction without redness and swelling of the overlying tissues and without increasing the patient's body temperature."(11)

Black recommended treating this ischemic osteonecrosis of the jawbone surgically, removing all bone until healthy bone filled in its place. His recommendations, however, and even his description of the disease, got lost somewhere in time.

The next mention of cavitations, as far as I can tell, appeared in a book called *Death and Dentistry*, written in 1940 by Martin Fischer, MD. The condition was observed by European physicians and dentists at the site of old extractions in the early 1950s. A decade later, articles began to appear in American medical and dental journals about cavitations, referring to them as "alveolar cavitational osteopathosis."

Bouquot reports that the dental profession did not rediscover the condition until the 1970s "when an unusual form of osteomyelitis of the jaw was noted in patients with chronic facial pain who were diagnosed with such conditions as atypical facial neuralgia/pain, trigeminal neuralgia, phantom toothache or headache."(12) Due to the absence of overt signs of infection/inflammation in tissue and on x-ray, the condition was referred to as "invisible osteomyelitis." Many other terms were subsequently used to describe cavitations. The most commonly used term today is NICO, Neuralgia-Inducing Cavitational Osteonecrosis. The term is somewhat misleading, since it implies that cavitations will cause neuralgia. Cavitations certainly *can* cause neuralgia – but not always. Instead, they can give rise to a variety of other systemic problems that would not likely be recognized as emanating from the jawbone.

The understanding of NICO (and its systemic effects) among medical and dental practitioners took a step forward in February, 1993, when a three-day symposium on the subject was held in California. Researchers presented studies and reports to doctors and dentists from all over the world, and a new awareness of the jawbone cavitation problem was born.

NECROSIS VS. MYELITIS

It is important to realize that the presence of bacteria in cavitation sites, albeit quite harmful, is secondary to the presence of avascular conditions which give rise to necrosis. It must also be recognized that the infection they cause is a low grade, sub-clinical one which would not be detected using standard diagnostic tools. Typically, few inflammatory cells are seen. As Bouquot observes, "The hallmark of acute inflammation, the neutrophil, is *hardly ever seen* within NICO lesions."(13)   Even if the silent infection *is* recognized, it is difficult to treat, due to the poor blood supply to the area. The avascular conditions would make it unlikely that antibiotics would reach the infection site. According to Meinig, some dentists believe antibiotic use may have the adverse effect of converting osteoblasts to osteocytes (which break down bone).(14)   Since blast cells generate new bone, antibiotics may therefore actually interfere with the healing process. Also, according to an Internet page on cavitations (http://www.hugnet.com/cavitati.htm), the real problem is not with bacteria at these sites, but rather, with the very strong chemicals they produce. These chemicals are "highly neurotoxic and kill many critical enzymes within the body." Since they are more of a problem than bacterial infection, antibiotic treatment of cavitations is considered (by Hal Huggins and associates) to be of "little value."

Dr. Christroher Hussar, DDS, DO, a specialist in cavitation surgery, has a different opinion on the use of antibiotics:

> *I believe antibiotics certainly have a place in cavitation surgery. Having performed this surgery for approximately ten years now, I find that patients who don't receive antibiotics, either oral and/or IV, often don't do as well as those patients who do receive them. I think one reason for this is because most of the patients suffering from this condition are so immune compromised that they need a certain amount of help to eradicate the residual bacterial infections that I believe are the primary cause for cavitations to exist.*

Although the use of antibiotics can often result in rather rapid symptom relief, that relief is accomplished in a manner which interrupts the body's healing mechanisms and therefore may cause more problems in the long run. Later on, through their action of symptom suppression, antibiotics may serve to drive toxins deeper into the system. The work of Hans Heinrich Reckweg, MD, as put forth in *Homotoxicology*, provides a scientific basis for such reasoning. Jack Tips, ND, Ph.D, offers this interesting insight on antibiotic use:

> *A few doctors are daring to think that perhaps antibiotics do not thoroughly kill infectious diseases, but only force the body to accept them and end the fight – a conditional surrender rather than a victory. From an energy perspective, antibiotics encourage bacteria to mutate or expand their rate of oscillation. This moves them into the realm of healthy oscillation, causing frequent problems – i.e., new varieties with greater activity in the human system. The suppression of bacteria (and the immune system) with antibiotics may have opened the door to the more detrimental viral involvements.*(15)

Personally, I try to avoid antibiotic use whenever possible. I will concede, however, that their *appropriate* use can save lives. Opinions differ, however, as to what is appropriate.

Even biological medicines injected directly into a must cavitation site cannot eradicate bacteria until the *conditions* giving rise to them are corrected. It is more technically correct, therefore, to view cavitations as an osteo*necrotic* condition, rather than an osteo*myeletic* one, although they may, in fact, be both and often are. We need to keep in mind that cavitations result from poor vascular circulation in the jaw. Bacterial involvement is secondary. Therefore, to be successful, treatment must focus *initially* on removal of disease conditions – periodontal ligament (if still present) and necrotic bone. This can only be accomplished surgically.

SURGICAL PROCEDURE

To avoid the development of cavitations following extraction, it is said to be necessary for the surgeon to remove the periodontal ligament and approximately one millimeter of the bony socket, as both bone and ligament are usually infected with bacteria. The cutting or "perturbing" of the bone also stimulates a cellular change from osteocytes to osteoblasts, aiding in new bone formation. This is usually a simple surgical procedure with new extractions. When dealing with healed-over sockets, however, the procedure is more involved and is complicated at the present time by limited availablity of reliable diagnostic apparatus that would allow the surgeon to pinpoint the exact location and dimensions of the cavitation(s).

Oral surgeon and osteopath, Christopher Hussar, has shared with me the very reasonable perspective that removal of more than one millimeter of the bony socket may, at times, be necessary.

> If you are going to do cavitational surgery, it is very important that you remove all diseased bone with your burr and/or manual instruments. You cannot designate a one millimeter goal. I have seen cavitations tower upwards of six centimeters. You must remove any and all diseased bone, as if you were a cancer surgeon removing a ror, in order for the immune system to get back on back to obtain some semblance of stren g component, namely cavitations.

DIAGNOSTIC LIMITATIONS

Cavitations do not always show up on x-ray. Even when radiographic indications *are* present, they can be difficult to spot for the untrained eye, since the changes are quite subtle and can easily be missed or misinterpreted. Thirty to fifty percent of the bone must be destroyed before it is visible on x-ray.(16)

In a properly done extraction (where the socket is cleaned out, with periodontal ligament and an appropriate amount of the bony socket removed), the outline of roots seen on x-ray will disappear within a year. However, according to Peter Brawn, DDS, "Five to ten years after tooth extraction... [presence of] the outline of the previous roots is a classic indication that there is a NICO lesion."(17) X -rays cannot be relied upon to rule out cavitations, however, for as Thomas Levy, MD (cavitations video) observes, it is "the exception, rather than the rule" for cavitations to show up on x-ray.

Dr. Chris Hussar has a different point of view, as expressed in a letter to me:

> *To the trained eye, most of the time, I would say within a 90% judgment, these cavitations are quite visible on x-ray, either from the bony tenure within them or the changes that exist surrounding the cavitation. These changes include destruction of the bony canal through which the major nerve of the lower jaw (the inferior alveolar nerve) courses. Usually you see the superior aspect of the canal destroyed by cavitation. The consistency and density of the bone will be different compared to surrounding bone. Oftentimes you will see microcalcifications which indicate the presence of a cavitation.*

Special sonogram equipment, approved as a research tool by the FDA for use in dentistry and designed to detect cavitations, was released at the end of 1999 and is now being used by a limited number of dentists and doctors. Use of this "Cavitat" machine, will no doubt spread. Such equipment will not only help surgeons locate the cavitations, but will yield information about their dimensions. Currently in limited use for locating the cavitations are alsoTech-99 bone scans, as well as thermography, which displays areas of both hot (infected) and cold (normal) bone (the CRT 2000 is an instrument which has been particularly useful in this regard). ElectroDermal Screening can also be used to locate cavitations and ascertain their connection to systemic disorders. This type of testing measures energy flow through channels (meridians) of the body in a non-invasive manner. It can yield impressive results, but can also miss some problem areas (as per my experience). Unless conducted by a qualified practitioner (often an acupuncture physician) who is aware of the tooth-body connection and special EDS dental screening protocols, this type of testing will fail to reveal the presence of jawbone cavitations. A skilled EDS practitioner can be a valuable asset to cavitation surgery. His or her instrument can provide feedback about the success of surgery as it is being performed. The Cavitat machine can serve this function as well. CAT scans and MRI have also been used to detect large jawbone cavitations.

Some dentists will use a "neural therapy anesthetic nerve block" diagnostically to find cavitations. With this technique they may check the body's response with applied kinesiology (muscle testing), looking for a muscle response that is weak when they "therapy localize" (connect energetically through touch) to the area of distress in the jaw, and then becomes strong when anesthesia is injected into that area. When the affected portion of the jawbone is thus electrically disconnected from the rest of the body (an effect of the anesthesia), symptoms elsewhere in the body related to that tooth's area in the mouth have often been observed to clear up, according to Los Angeles dentist, Harold Ravins.(18) Hidden infections in intact teeth can be located in like manner. The energetic relationship between teeth and body organs is illustrated on the chart in Appendix A.

Bouquot describes the cavitation site as a "small zone of hyperesthesia or normal pain response in an area otherwise (numbed by) local anesthesia."(19) When I read these words, it brought to mind the difficulty my surgeon had getting my upper jaw numbed at the cavitation sites. Another statement of Bouquot's explained why extractions and some of my crown replacements done over the years have been so painful: "The local deficit [in blood flow] does not allow the affected jawbone to respond normally to routine dental work and/or bone infections or to trauma such as tooth extraction."(20)

Due to a long-standing dearth of reliable diagnostic equipment to detect cavitations, many dentists have relied upon their drill and sense of touch to locate these jawbone pockets. Typically they will drill small holes into the jawbone at various spots along the sites of old extractions. When they go in above a cavitation site, the drill will drop through the soft bone into the hole. This feels vastly different than when they drill into solid bone. Crude though this technique may be, it seems to be a widely used one. It is one with which Dr. Hussar takes issue, however, believing that "this type of punching through the jawbone without a flap and using just a burr is highly incorrect and does more harm than good." Dr. Hussar has expressed very candidly to me his belief that there are "only perhaps a handful of people in the entire country that are doing cavitational surgery correctly" at this time. There is quite a difference between just drilling a hole in the jawbone and irrigating with an antiseptic solution, and doing full flap surgery, where an actual surgical incision is made in the gum tissue. Look for a dentist trained in the latter. Dr. Wesley Shankland, DDS, MS, PhD, another expert in cavitation surgery, agrees with this advice. In his words:

> A surgical site <u>must</u> be operated via an incision, reflection of a flap, removal of the outside bone (cortical plate) in order to "see" the extent of the lesion. This procedure has to be followed. No exceptions.

TREATMENT OUTCOMES

The success of cavitation surgery appears to have been measured thus far by the yardstick of relief of facial pain. This would not appear to be a particularly reliable yardstick, not only because of its subjective nature, but also due largely to the fact that cavitations often (more often than not) cause no local pain. Nonetheless, the only statistics to which I currently have access are based on this criterion. Drs. Bennett and Brawn report that 60% of patients recover completely following surgical treatment and 14% have "mild, occasional pain."(21) Presumably then, 26% experience no improvement.

Bouquot reports a 70% overall cure rate (with "freedom from pain" for approximately five years being the criterion for cure).(22)   He observes, as have others, that there is a strong tendency for cavitations to recur and for new ones to develop. Thus repetition of the surgical procedure, sometimes numerous times, can be necessary. Bouquot notes that 80% of NICO patients who fail to respond after their initial surgery have some sort of clotting disorder.(23)

Clotting problems or other vascular abnormalities also may *predispose* one to cavitation problems. When a good blood clot doesn't form and remain intact following tooth extraction, the result is a painful condition called a "dry socket." According to Frank Jerome, DDS, author of *Tooth Truth*, "The tooth sites most likely to form cavitations are the wisdom teeth *and* any extractions that turn into a dry socket."(24)

The poor bone healing so many cavitation patients seem to experience following surgery may be due in part to decreased levels of calcium and phosphorus in the affected areas of the jawbone. The reason for these deficiencies is unknown.

Thomas Levy, MD suggests that cavitations could accurately be described as pockets of necrosis or *intraosseous gangrene*. As gangrene has a tendency to spread, so do cavitations. According to Dr. Michael LaMarche:

> *It [the cavitation] can actually destroy a blood vessel and through the channel that the blood vessel courses, the cavitation can grow and can include a number of teeth or areas of former teeth. It can grow that way, so we find a tunneling. When we open into one, we find that actually the one becomes two becomes three, and as many as four or five of the formerly extracted teeth. Sometimes these will go around teeth that we believe to be vital.*(25)

The spreading of cavitations very likely constitutes a major overlooked cause of tooth loss. To my knowledge, factors which trigger the spreading have not yet been identified, but they would no doubt encompass those known to initiate them in the first place. (See lists on subsequent pages.) In my own case, spreading seemed to have been promoted by placement of incompatible metals in my mouth near a major cavitation site. More on that later.

When cavitations spread, they do so in an almost imperceptible manner, forming small "wormhole" connections between adjacent sites. It is also possible for the diameter of the original cavitation to expand to encompass the area of one or more tooth sites, as Dr. LaMarche describes above. In the case of the small wormholes, it is possible they remain in whole or in part following surgery. Their presence may be a factor in recurrence of cavitations and return of symptoms, though admittedly this is strictly my speculation – the ruminations of a professional dental patient!

Bouquot suggests that a patient's prognosis for recovery may be improved by combining surgery with hyberbaric oxygen therapy. He also believes that the use of various anti-clotting therapies may prove to be beneficial. Dr. Thomas Levy recommends use of an intravenous infusion of vitamin C during surgery to assist in detoxification, as well as the use of north pole magnetic energy afterward to control pain and promote healing.(26)

In dealing with systemic infection emanating from oral foci, the issue of mercury toxicity must be addressed. If you have amalgam in your mouth, it must be *properly* removed (see Dr. Huggins' book, *Detoxification*, for details).

If your amalgam has been replaced with composite or ceramic material – even if the replacement was done years ago – it is quite likely you are still retaining mercury in your tissues. This heavy metal will not leave the body unless a good detoxification program is being followed. Even then, its departure is very slow.

Failure to detoxify the body of mercury can result in perpetuation of systemic infection. Here's why: Mercury kills cells by suffocating them. The body therefore cultivates bacteria and fungi so that the metal will instead cling to *their* cell walls – i.e., the body chooses infection over mercury-induced cell death. To attempt to rid the body of bacteria or fungi without detoxifying it of mercury will therefore be unsuccessful in the long run. I believe this may be why so many people have trouble getting rid of candida infections, even when faithfully following an anti-candida treatment. The conditions of mercury toxicity and cavitations must first be addressed.

Hair analysis is one tool for detecting mercury toxicity; although the problem may not surface if the metal is being retained in storage sites. Electro Dermal Screening (EDS) can also pick up mercury toxicity, as can Applied Kinesiology in some instances. Additionally, urine (porphyrin) and fecal analyses can be used to detect heavy metals.

For more information on mercury toxicity and detoxi-fication, contact DAMS, Inc. (Dental Amalgam Mercury Survivors), P.O. Box 7249 Minneapolis, MN 55407-0249, or toll-free: 1-800-311-6265. The Environmental Dental Association (1-800-388-8124) can also provide information, as well as a list of qualified practitioners.

A very informative website dealing with this issue is Dr. Deborah Baker's www.y2khealthanddetox.com. Dr. Baker recommends the use of specific nutrients, including vitamins C and E, glutathione, N-Acetyl-Cysteine, Alpha-lipoic acid and selenium to assist the body with mercury detoxification by supporting the liver. She cautions against the potentially devastating effects of the popular chemical chelator, DMPS, which include mercury redistribution. She also advises great care with the use of orally administered DMSA which can remove mercury from the brain, but can also remove nutrient minerals from the body.

STATISTICS

Nobody knows for sure exactly how often routine extractions result in the formation of cavitations. Estimates run as high as 80-90%. The farther back in the mouth the extraction site, the greater the likelihood of problems occurring. Thomas Levy, MD quotes studies done in conjunction with Hal Huggins which reveal a 77% overall incidence of cavitations (536 of 691 extraction sites) and an 85% incidence in 3rd molars (wisdom teeth).(27)   He adds that this is considered an *under*estimate, owing to present day diagnostic limitations. Bouquot has found that wisdom teeth sites constitute about 45% of all jawbone cavitations. His biopsies confirm the presence of cavitations in one of every 2,200 - 5,000 adults – that is more than 68,000 American adults. Bouquot notes that the condition has been diagnosed in patients ranging from 16-94 years of age, both male and female. The preponderance of cases, however, occur in females (75%) between the ages of 35 and 64 (71%). He goes on to state, "One-third of patients have more than a single quadrant involved and 10% have lesions in all four quadrants, not necessarily at the same time."(28)

Dr. Hussar has made the following statement to me regarding the extent of the cavitation problem:

> *Through sheer numbers alone you have to assume that the cavitational problem is indeed epidemic. With over thousands of biopsies performed over a period of several years, I have had probably two or three normal bone tissue reports returned. Therefore, with a 98-99% accuracy, one can assume that cavitations are present.*

OTHER CAUSES

Thus far I have mentioned only extractions as a cause of jawbone cavitations. Although it is undoubtedly accurate to say they are the *major* cause, it should be noted that other conditions can also give rise to the devel- opment of cavitations. Other factors and/or conditions with which cavitations have an *established* strong association, according to Bouquot, who extrapolated from the literature on hip osteonecrosis, are:

- Other oral surgery or localized trauma
- Endodontic therapy
- Cushing's Syndrome (a disease caused by overproduction of cortisone)
- Corticosteroid therapy (both long and short term)
- Radiation therapy for cancer
- Variable atmospheric pressures (occurring in some occupations)
- Alcoholism
- Systemic Lupus Erythematosus
- Sickle Cell Anemia
- Pancreatitis
- Thrombophilia (Protein C and Protein S deficiencies)
- Gaucher's Disease
- Familial Hypofibrinolysis Disease (plasminogen inhibitor deficiency)[29]

There is also a strong, but as yet unproven, association between cavitations and intraosseous (inside the bone) inflammation and infection. Bouquot observes that "recurrent sinusitis may cause destruction of bony walls and floor of the maxillary sinus, thereby allowing bacteria and/or inflammatory toxins into alveolar [jaw]bone on a recurring basis."[30]   He also notes that root canal fillings which are causing pain to the patient, despite looking normal on x-ray, can be a source of infection and therefore serve as a trigger in the formation of cavitations. According to Michael G. LaMarche, DDS, one of 30 members of the North American Research Group formed by Dr. Bouquot, 147 of 150 of the root canal-filled teeth removed by dentists in his group were found to have ischemic osteonecrosis around the tooth.(31) It is important to note, however, that jawbone cavitations have been found in patients *without* extractions, root canal fillings or sinusitis. With these patients, one or more of the above factors may serve as a trigger – and/or one or more of those listed below. With those below there is again a strong, though unproven, association with cavitation development, as per Bouquot:

- Rheumatoid arthritis
- Prosthetic obstruction of blood flow to marrow
- Intraosseous malignancy (especially lymphoma and metastatic carcinoma)
- Pregnancy/high dose estrogen therapy
- Antiphospholipid Antibody Syndrome
- Cigarette smoking
- Disseminated Intravascular Coagulation (DIC) (32)

Although there are causes other than tooth extraction for cavitation formation, the problem remains *primarily* an iatrogenic (physician-induced, or in this case, dentist-induced) one. Many dedicated and skilled oral surgeons and dentists are unknowingly inflicting a great deal of suffering upon their patients by employing faulty extraction protocol: i.e., not removing the entire periodontal ligament and an appropriate portion of the bony socket. It is imperative that these practitioners be educated about the health hazards posed by cavitations and how they can be avoided.

THE "WISDOM" OF REMOVING WISDOM TEETH

Most of us have had our wisdom teeth removed, either because we had problems or because it was feared they might cause future problems. These problems and potential ones stem from the fact that most of us just don't have room for these 3rd molars in our jaws. They are too narrow. This has led to the theory that the human race has evolved beyond the need for wisdom teeth, that our narrow jaws are an evolutionary adaptation which obviates the need for 3rd molars. Such scholarly speculation is nonsense. The widespread incidence of narrow dental arches seen in civilized cultures is nothing more than the result of toxic damage and deficiency caused by poor diet.

Dr. Weston Price, the dentist who did the pioneering root canal research earlier in this century, proved this conclusively through epidemiological (population) studies. During the 1930s, Price and his wife embarked upon a ten-year research project in which every summer they visited a different place in the world where the inhabitants were still eating their native diet. The Prices studied 14 different races of people who did not have access to the foods of modern civilization. Dr. Price made meticulous notes on the oral and general health of these natives and compiled his data and conclusions in *Nutrition and Physical Degeneration*.

He found that the rate of tooth decay among these people was very low – less than 5% compared to the 90%+ among our people. He attributed the difference in decay rate to the difference in diet. These natives ate a variety of natural foods and their diets contained no sugar or white flour. They consumed whole foods containing an abundance of fat-soluble vitamins (A,D,E,F), ten times more than we consume today in our culture. The amount of water-soluble vitamins (B,C) and minerals in their diet was likewise greater, by at least four times.

Significantly, Price found that the natives who ate their traditional diets had *broad facial structures and straight teeth*. Their wide dental arches could easily support 3rd molars.

Price also examined tribe members who had been in contact with the outside world and had begun consuming its white sugar and flour products. He found that, not only did these individuals develop extensive tooth decay, but *their children were born with narrow jaws . . .and their teeth came in crooked.* Price demonstrated conclusively that **a poor diet can alter basic bone structure in just one generation.**

Thus, we who are products of multiple generations of "civilized" living and eating are heirs to narrow dental arches that will not accommodate wisdom teeth. This being the case, removal of these teeth may indeed be necessary. However, if the surgeon removing your 3rd molars does not properly clean the socket, you will be at higher risk for more problems later. If your wisdom teeth are long gone, you can be sure there is an extremely high probability the proper procedure was not followed for their removal – because it was unknown to your dentist. If you then later lose other teeth, even if their sockets *are* properly cleaned out, cavitations from the old 3rd molar sites can easily spread to these new sites and beyond. For this reason *it is absolutely necessary to correct cavitation problems in healed-over extraction sites,* in addition to assuring that sockets of newly extracted teeth are properly cleaned at the time of surgery.

Cavitations often occur in the retromolar area (beyond the wisdom teeth sites in the mandible). The body tends to stash toxins here, especially heavy metals and parasite toxins, according to acupuncturist, Doug Leber, who believes this may be done by the body in an effort to protect the brain. When the holding capacity of the retromolar areas has been exceeded, toxins spill over into weakened areas of the body.

THE TOOTH-BODY CONNECTION

The association between cavitations and facial pain such as trigeminal neuralgia, has already been touched upon, as well as phantom toothache and headaches. Other conditions that have resolved for some people following cavitation surgery include heart murmur, multiple sclerosis, food sensitivities, balance and eye problems.(33)

Dr. Hussar describes a patient who for years had eye pain and double vision that was unresponsive to standard medical treatment. Two months after surgical treatment of four cavitations, this woman reported being pain-free and able to read for the first time in years.(34)   Dr. Hussar also tells the story of an 85-year old woman with knee pain so intense she couldn't wear stockings. After surgical treatment of cavitations, she "was dancing around the room."

In *Root Canal Cover Up*, Dr. Meinig describes two cases in which the patients experienced complete remission of all symptoms following surgical treatment of cavitations. One was a woman who suffered from migraine headaches almost every day for three years, "a variety of intestinal and stomach upsets," and severe sinus problems. The other was a man who had spent $13,000 on medical treatment and continued to suffer from arthritis of the knee and leg. He was pain-free the day after cavitation surgery.(35)

Such rapid remission of symptoms following surgery sometimes occurs, but not always. In some cases, response is less rapid, presumably because the body needs time to rid itself of accumulated toxins and heal the damage caused by them. In other cases, surgical treatment of cavitations in itself is insufficient. An aggressive detoxification program is also needed. Cavitations in the jawbone, particularly long-standing ones, can be a fountain from which toxins are continually spewing. Although surgery may turn off the fountain, thus halting the toxin flow, it does not mop up toxic residues that may have permeated the system. Remember: The toxins from bacteria in cavitations are some of the deadliest known. It can be a challenge to rid the body of these super toxins. Finding an effective way to do so is the subject of on-going research. Toxicology studies performed on tissue samples can provide important clues to adjunctive therapies that may produce results.

Not all patients treated for cavitations have a successful recovery. Dr. LaMarche describes the case of a man who suffered from the intense pain of trigeminal neuralgia.(36) This man had all of his teeth removed many years prior to having cavitation surgery at three upper extraction sites. The surgery did successfully eliminate the pain. However, it returned after five years and became so intense that the man committed suicide. He willed his skull to Dr. Bouquot for research purposes, and autopsy revealed spreading of the jawbone cavitations. Study of this skull has helped advance cavitation research considerably.

Virtually any organ or body system can be adversely affected by the presence of jawbone cavitations. That chronic degenerative disease of such organs as kidneys, liver, stomach or brain can have its etiology (origin) in the jawbone is a foreign idea to most people in our culture, lay persons and professionals alike. Nonetheless, it is an idea that has been around for a long time and has impressive research to back it up.

THE FOCAL INFECTION THEORY

About 40 years ago, Patrick Störtebecker, MD, Ph.D, presented evidence of the systemic spread of microorganisms and their toxins from osteitis-affected jawbone through cranial venous pathways, the trigeminal nerve and other cranial nerves.[37]

Störtebecker's studies established a link between root canal infections and the following disorders: brain cancer, multiple sclerosis, encephalitis, epilepsy, schizophrenia, Alzheimer's and Parkinson's diseases, disease of the eyes, jaw, mouth and throat. Other research has linked root canals to a number of other disorders, including "kidney, liver and gall bladder problems, back, neck and shoulder pain, eye, ear and skin conditions, neuritis, neuralgia, appendicitis, pneumonia, rheumatism, shingles, arthritis, stomach ulcers, ovarian cysts, testicle infections, intestinal problems and Attention Deficit/Hyperactivity Disorder."[38]

The spread of toxins throughout the system, whether from root canals or cavitations, appears to follow the same principles and pathways. In both cases, it begins with microbial invasion of the bone and spreads via pathways described by Störtebecker. Therefore, all of the conditions listed above (and more) can result from cavitations as well as root canals.

According to Störtebecker, bacteria in the jaw can produce enough poison to make the blood pressure go up: "A highly common oral microbe, streptococcus faecalis, can produce tyramine, a vasopressor substance [raises blood pressure]. Many of the people walking around with high blood pressure have dental infections. And nobody will look at the teeth."(39)

Störtebecker also makes a fascinating connection between microorganisms found in the jawbone and brain cancer:

> There are many cases observed of fungus in the brain associated with brain tumors. Nobody comments that molds and common bacteria, such as e. coli, have the capacity to synthesize complex cyclic hydrocarbons, i.e., potent carcinogens. In one case, a 25-year old man had a history of pain on the right side of his face. In the first surgical procedure, there was no tumor, only a ray fungus the size of a nut.
>
> Screening to locate the primary site of the infection revealed a bone inflammation of the same-sided "wisdom tooth." When a culture was taken, it grew the same microorganism (actinomyces Israeli) that was found in the brain. Half a year later the patient died and there wasn't any ray fungus left, but only a malignant tumor, big as an apple. A very famous scientist was quite convinced that the ray fungus had produced the tumor. But at that time (1940), we didn't know the ray fungus could produce carcinogenic substances. That was only in the 50s and 60s. Even today, doctors say cases like this are just a coincidence. They just don't understand.(40)

You'd think they *would* understand, for as Meinig observes, dentists are taught that they must prescribe antibiotics before and after treatment (or even simple cleanings) to patients with a history of certain cardiac problems. They do this in order to prevent endocarditis, an infectious condition — a *focal* infection if coming from the mouth!(41)

The jawbone, along with the teeth, gums and tonsils, represents an area of the body which frequently serves as a focus of infection. A "focus" is a walled-off area of concentrated toxins where necrotic tissue and/or infection can be found. It is a form of "interference field" that blocks the energy flow through any acupuncture meridians (energy channels) going through it. Since the meridians supply energy to distant organs and many of them run through the head, a focus there can cause numerous systemic conditions. Scars, electrical currents and toxic metals, as well as foci, can create fields of disturbance, having a profound effect upon the entire body.

THE SIGNIFICANCE OF HEAD FOCI

In a paper entitled *More Cures for Cancer,* translated from German, the late Dr. Med. Josef Issels wrote of the significance of these focal infections in systemic disorders: "Unquestionable facts gathered from long medical and dental experience show clearly the direct relation between general disorders and hidden chronic focus in the head."[42] He lists the following disorders as those "demonstrably proved to be partly caused by the presence of non-eliminated focus:"

- rheumatic disorders
- urogenital disorders
- renal (kidney) disorders
- opthalmologic disorders
- dermatologic disorders
- asthma
- cardiovascular disorders
- multiple sclerosis
- gastrointestinal disorders
- epilepsy

Although focal infection theory is alien to most doctors and dentists in the U.S., the German Medical Association for Focal Research routinely informs members of the medical and dental professions of progress in international research on this important subject. This organization defines focus as "an abnormally localized alteration in the organism, with the capacity to induce distant actions out of its immediate proximity."[43]

In the focal theory, any chronic inflammation, scar or degenerative condition in the body can be an active focus or "interference field." Issels tells us that the focus is "embedded in the *mesenchymal* base tissue."(44)   Mesenchyme is defined as "loosely organized mesodermal cells that give rise to such structures as connective tissues, blood, lymphatics, bone and cartilage." Because of its mesenchymal roots, the focus has direct contact with blood and lymphatic circulation, as well as what Issels refers to as "neuro-vegetative nerve fiber." This connection to mesenchymal tissue forms the vehicle through which the focus spreads to the rest of the body.

Issels states that whether or not a focus expresses itself in "distant actions in the organism" depends upon the organism's local defense mechanism. He is very clear about the focal effects of root canals, quoting Schondorf: "A root canal treatment which does not plant a focus *does not exist.*"(45)   The root canal-filled tooth is described as a "toxin factory which continually damages the organism." However, since no pain is felt in the avital tooth, the patient is unaware of the toxic focus which will continue to "unfold its devastating effect for decades and quite often for a lifetime. The inflammatory process ultimately spreads to the jawbone, causing osteomyelitis" – and cavitations!

There are basically four ways in which a dental focus can affect the organism, according to Issels: **neural, toxic, allergic** and **bacterial.** Neural therapy can only be successful in eliminating the *neural* effects of a focus. Toxic and allergic effects must be addressed through the elimination of the focus. According to Issels, "The toxic effect of the dental focus seems to be even more significant for the whole organism than the neural effect of the disturbance."(46)

Focal toxins are described as "organic or anorganic matter which are neither detoxified by the organism nor broken down with inflammatory reactions. They are therefore often stored in the connective tissue."(47)   Issels observed that patients with dental and tonsillar foci were found to have significantly increased blood levels of di-methyl-sulphur. This substance is closely related to the poison gases used in combat during World War I in terms of both structure and effect. Elimination of foci has been demonstrated to return blood levels of di-methyl-sulphur to normal.

Circulating toxins play a role in allergicly sensitizing the organism through their interaction with proteins.

The bacterial effect of dental foci is generally asymptomatic, but can result in the formation of a "secondary focus," often in the sinuses, gall bladder, appendix, prostate or renal pelvis.(48)

Issels describes hospital tests which he conducted that confirmed a causal relationship between presence of foci in the head and tumor development elsewhere in the body. Infrared radiation, which increases in intensity on the skin surface of an area of "inflammatory pathogenous focus," was used in the studies.(49)   Issels states quite bluntly that the role of dental and tonsillar foci is so pronounced in cancer that he considers it *malpractice* to overlook this factor in therapy.

THE TONSILLAR FOCUS

Issels tells us that "chronic inflamed tonsils are the primary focus of the head which frequently can have a more severe effect for the whole organism than the dental focus."(50)   His tests with infrared radiation have shown the relation of tonsillar focus to tumor activity.

Issels describes a "degenerative-atrophic tonsillitis" which is characterized by small tonsils, lack of inflammation and tenacious attachment to their bed. These types of degenerated tonsils, frequently found in the cancer patient, "can no longer detoxify and have become . . . a most dangerous toxic focus. As with nerve avital teeth and other dental focus, they must be removed."(51)   Issels has noted significant improvement in cancer patients following tonsillectomy and elimination of dental foci.

It should be noted that toxins from dental foci can and will invade the tonsils (or stubs of the tonsils where the organ has been surgically removed). Therefore, elimination of tonsillar foci should logically follow elimination of dental foci. Where a tonsillectomy has already been performed, the toxic focus remaining in the stub of the tonsils can be addressed with a neural therapy technique involving injection of the area (with an anesthetic or with a biological medicine), along with manual manipulation of the tissue. This same technique can be used with intact tonsils.

Not withstanding the established benefits of neural therapy, I believe the use of aniline based local anethetics should be limited due to their demonstrated neurotoxicity and carcinogenic effects. Aniline based anethetics are those whose names end in "caine," such as lidocaine.

CHAPTER FIVE

MY TOOTH/BODY CONNECTION

I've often said that someday I'm going to write a book called *Never the Same Since* — in recognition of the fact that many people go through life seemingly well until falling victim to some illness or injury from which they never fully recover. For me that event took place in 1983 when I developed an aberrant breathing pattern as the result of an injury months earlier involving my upper torso. It took five years to resolve the problem, after which time I was symptom-free for another five years – until I began extensive dental treatment which started with the simple replacement of a crown. After that crown replacement I began to re-experience breathing, as well as old bladder problems (which had originally manifested as infection when I was young and as "interstitial cystitis," an "incurable" bladder condition, after the injury of '82.)

It took me a long time to realize that the problems were related to my mouth. Having had my amalgams removed in '83, I was confident I had taken the necessary steps to avert any dentally induced systemic illness. I was wrong. My first clue that the systemic problems were indeed related to hidden dental ones came in 1994 when bladder symptoms of one year duration were completely resolved after the extraction of a tooth. Unfortunately, that tooth was replaced with a bridge made of the same metallic (though mercury-free) material of which the aforementioned replace-ment crown was made. My bladder symptoms returned after that. Following placement of the above mentioned crown, I entered a *dental hell* from which I am only now emerging. For the entire period of time I was plagued with old – and new – health problems, and I also lost six more teeth, one at a time. In retrospect, I can say that what appears to have happened is that the toxins from the metals in the crown and bridge material triggered the spreading of already existing cavitations caused by old extractions.

Like most people, I lost my wisdom teeth (third molars) early in life, having all four extracted soon after they came in, in the name (ironically) of "*preventing* future problems."

I wouldn't lose another tooth until 1992 when the lower right second molar started hurting me for no apparent reason. I would later learn, however, that this tooth's former neighbor, the previously extracted third molar, was not *completely* extracted: A piece of the root remained lodged in my jawbone. I can see now that this root fragment posed a formidable barrier to healing of the socket, allowing for development of a cavitation of substantial size which would spread rapidly. This affected other teeth, after a metal crown and bridge were placed in my otherwise metal-free mouth.

THE ROLE OF MATERIALS

It took awhile after my body began malfunctioning and I began losing my teeth one by one for me to realize that cavitations might be the culprit. By then I had already identified and replaced all incompatible composite materials which had much earlier replaced amalgams. This was a lengthy and expensive process that literally bankrupted me, but I was willing to do it because I thought it would make me well. It didn't. In fact, the trauma of the dental work probably caused spreading of cavitations. In retrospect, I can say, although it is *vitally important* to replace incompatible materials, both metallic and nonmetallic, it is equally important to identify and treat cavitations. Material compatibility can be established through blood testing (Clifford or Huggins) available through most mercury-free dentists. ElectroDermal Screening can also be used. Using both methods when possible is ideal.

SURGERY NECESSARY

After finally realizing cavitations were causing my problems, I looked for a dentist who could treat them. Finding one was difficult, but I managed to locate one some distance from me. He used a variation of "neural therapy," involving a 'stabident' procedure, wherein a small hole was drilled into the jawbone through which biological medicines (Sanum remedies) were injected to treat the infection. Unfortunately, I would eventually come to realize that this treatment was a *total failure* at correcting the cavitation problem. Worse yet, it appeared to have cost me the loss of yet another tooth. The reason for this failure is now apparent to me: It sought to treat the element of *infection* associated with the cavitations while doing nothing to correct the *conditions* giving rise to that infection and perpetuating it – namely, presence of any remnants of the periodontal ligament and/or necrotic bone tissue. Neither the ligament (if still present), nor the necrotic bone, can be eliminated through non-surgical treatment, as I've discussed.   The presence of either or both creates conditions favorable to the proliferation of anaerobic bacteria. The bacteria, however, are not the original problem. They are the *result* of it. Therefore, although I am not a great fan of surgery, in the case of cavitations, I see no viable alternative. The use of Sanum injections *post*operatively – in both jawbone and tonsils – *may* be useful in eliminating toxic residues, but their use will *not* obviate the need for surgery. This is my opinion based upon my experience.

Although the kinesiology (muscle testing) used by practitioners of neural therapy in dentistry may prove useful in localizing cavitations, this process is a highly subjective one and can fail, as it did with me. I had been told during my final visit with the dentist who had been treating me non-surgically over an eight-month period with Sanum injections and other therapies that "the cavitation areas were not testing at that point" (meaning no treatment of them was indicated based on muscle testing). Soon after this pronouncement, eleven cavitations, some of substantial size and interconnecting, were revealed by the dentist who did my surgery. (See photos in Appendix C, taken in July, 1997 by the dentist.) Tissue samples taken from these cavitation sites were found to be "extremely toxic."(See toxicology reports in Appendix B)

WHY ME?

I have speculated about why cavitations have caused me so much suffering, while other people who have them appear to be totally asymptomatic. I think the answer lies largely in the injury I sustained in 1982, the one from which I was "never the same since." Before then, my body was successfully managing to seal off and contain the bacteria and their toxins present in extraction sites (at that point only the wisdom teeth areas). After the injury, containment was no longer possible, since energy was diverted to deal with the new trauma. It appears that the body works on a priority basis, and I had developed a new priority. Still my body managed to contain the cavitations to some degree for another ten years, since I did not lose another tooth until 1992. However, in the year that followed, when the incompatible metallic crown was placed in my mouth, cavitations began to spread, causing more tooth loss, as well as the return of old systemic problems. When a bridge of the same material was placed right next to the buried root fragment, the process accelerated, causing more tooth loss and more health problems. My condition continued to worsen – until my first cavitation surgery in the summer of 1997.

One answer as to why some people's cavitations spread rapidly and cause a great deal of systemic damage, and other people feel little or no effect from theirs, lies in the individual's medical history. Those who have been immune compromised through serious injury or illness are more likely to feel the full effects of their cavitations. No doubt the same can be said about those with an inherently weak constitution. The other factor I mentioned, the connection with metal dental materials, is at this time only my own observation. However, I feel confident that research will confirm the link between toxins from these metal materials and the forming and/or spreading of cavitations. Other variables, observed by Levy, are the amount of periodontal ligament left in the mouth after extraction and the particular microorganisms trapped at that time in the cavitation site.

Although usually no effort is made to remove the ligament during surgery, some portion (about half, according to Huggins) will automatically come out. If you are among those fortunate enough to have this membrane largely removed, the chances for a cavitation to form are minimal. Or, if one does, it will be benign in its effect. However, if a substantial portion of this ligament is left behind, it cannot be resorbed by the body, due to the avascular conditions. Since its presence forms a barrier to new bone growth, a cavitation will most certainly form. And aerobic bacteria will most certainly become trapped in this anaerobic environment, causing them to mutate and giving rise to the production of potent toxins – just how potent depends upon which particular bacteria become trapped. Again, it is a matter of chance.

In my case, I have no way of knowing how much of the periodontal ligament was left after my wisdom teeth were extracted over twenty years ago, but I do know a large amount of root was left at one site. This situation, along with my history of illness and injury and the subsequent placement and replacement (trauma) of incompatible metals (toxins) and other materials, set the stage for the development of a significant cavitation problem.

NOT THE SAME, BUT BETTER

Immediately following my first cavitation surgery, a tremendous amount of tension left my body. That was the first thing I noticed. Within days, chronic neck and shoulder pain subsided completely. My energy level and strength increased substantially. The two chronic health problems – bladder and breathing – did not resolve, however. Since my body was so extremely toxic from numerous cavitations of long standing, I was not among those who have been fortunate enough to experience immediate and complete remission of *all* symptoms following surgery. It was a blessing, however, to be rid of *some* of them.

As the cavitations were cleaned out, tissue samples were taken from all four quadrants of my mouth and submitted for biopsy and toxicology studies. The biopsies rule out malignancy, can tell if evidence of infection is present and may identify microorganisms. The toxicology reports give information on the toxins produced by the bacteria. Since these have not yet been conclusively identified, the report is limited to reflecting *enzyme damage* done by these toxins. Efforts are ongoing to identify the toxins and find a way to treat them. My reports are reproduced in Appendix B. You will note there is one report for each quadrant of the mouth, a total of four biopsy reports and four toxicology reports. Also included is technical information on enzyme activity which explains the relationship between enzyme inhibition and level of toxicity.

Since toxins interfere with *porphyrin* metabolism, urinary porphyrin testing can also be used to assess the degree of toxicity in the body. High levels of this chemical (which is involved in energy production) will be excreted when the body is carrying a toxic burden from heavy metals, root canals and/or cavitations. Removal of these sources will result in a significant reduction of urinary porphyrin excretion. Thus, as Huggins suggested, "Monitoring the excretion of porphyrins in the urine is a good way to measure the success of treatment"(52) – whether it is amalgam replacement, root canal removal or cavitation surgery.

A year after my first surgery, a second was performed, after a scan on an early experimental model of the Cavitat machine indicated poor bone healing in my jaw. During the course of the second surgery, a bone growth protein was placed in the jawbone to encourage regeneration. My symptoms continued following surgery, however, and ultimately a third surgery was performed. This one was done in concert with the use of intravenous ultraviolet irradiation of the blood in the hope that the effect would be eradication of pathogens and accelerated bone healing. Unfortunately, a Cavitat scan done in late 1999 still showed incomplete bone healing. Poor bone healing is the challenge many have faced following cavitation surgery, especially those with long-standing problems. Although I apparently didn't benefit significantly from the use of this therapy, there are reports of others having experienced satisfying results. The quest continues for a solution to the cavitation problem.

A DENTAL DILEMMA

Generally we look to our dentists and other doctors for solutions to our dental and other health problems, and for answers to our questions. We expect them to know the answers and to have the solutions. Unfortunately, when it comes to cavitations, they are not likely to have even heard of them. Not only are most dentists without a solution to this problem, they are unaware of its existence – and the role they have played in creating it. What they don't know CAN HURT US!

It can be difficult to find a dentist who is part of the solution rather than part of the problem. It had been my intention in this book to provide the names, addresses and phone numbers of key dentists practicing cavitation surgery. However, before the manuscript was completed, I realized that to do so could jeopardize the work of these pioneering dentists. I have learned, through personal experience and research, that cavitation surgery is viewed by standard dentistry, in general, and endodontics, in particular, as unnecessary and questionable — even unethical. Why they so view it, in the face of overwhelming evidence of its efficacy, is not difficult to figure out. The situation is analogous to that of mercury and root canals: The dental organizations are not about to publicly acknowledge the problems created by these – or cavitations, for to do so would invite an avalanche of malpractice suits. Instead, these powerful and influential organizations seek to discredit the researchers, practitioners and writers who are daring to reveal the truth on the subject. The American Endodontic Association's reaction to all the "rumblings" about root canals and cavitations has been to brand the rumblers as "quacks" and launch an aggressive campaign against them and their work. In the 6/96 edition of their journal, the *Communique*, the American Association of Endodontists stated ". . . The practice of recommending the extraction of endontically treated teeth for the prevention of NICO, or any other disease, is unethical and should be reported immediately to the appropriate state board of dentistry."

One of the major purposes of writing this book is to deliver the message that most people have cavitations, but no symptoms – at least not in the mouth. You will not know what role, if any, cavitations are playing in your systemic disorders until you have them surgically treated, or at least diagnosed. In either case, a visit to a dentist versed in cavitation pathology is in order. If your systemic problems *do* have their origin in your mouth, no amount of symptomatic treatment will solve the problem. You can fast until the cows come home and follow all kinds of detoxification and nutrition programs. However, until you *shut off the toxin fountain in your jawbone*, you are not likely to take a significant step toward wellness. This has been my experience. If you wait until you are in crisis to do something about your cavitations, it is going to be a long road back to health. I know. I am on that road.

It is important to understand that the symptoms I have, as a result of cavitations, are unique to me. A number of people, perhaps a majority, will be totally asymptomatic – at least for a time. Others will display a wide variety of symptoms.

Symptoms may well be absent when the clinical picture is one of necrosis only, with no overtones of infection. Even where infection is present, if it has not yet gained systemic access, the individual will most likely be asymptomatic.

In the case of those individuals with chronic osteo-myelitis, where infection has gained access to the rest of the system, virtually any symptom or set of symptoms can result. Exactly what the symptoms will be will depend largely upon the person's inherent weaknesses and prior injuries and illnesses. Toxins tend to settle in the organs of greatest weakness. In my case, I developed bladder problems (a congenital weakness) and breathing problems of a neurological nature (from my "never the same since" injury of '82). For another person, cavitations will result in an entirely different symptom picture, one that is unique to that individual.

If you are fortunate enough to have no symptoms, *it does not mean you have no cavitations.* Most likely you do if you have had extractions, and chances are good that, with time, they will result in symptoms somewhere in your body. Therefore, it is the better part of wisdom to treat these cavitations now, before symptoms do develop, since added body stresses increase the spreading of toxicity. And early treatment increases the chance of full recovery.

Once you get into a situation like mine where super toxins have invaded the system, surgery will lessen the body's toxic burden. However, it will not wholly repair the damage. As yet, there is no definitive answer about how to make these repairs. In fact, we are still trying to figure out just *what* we're dealing with. Researchers are still working on identification of toxins present in cavitations.

SOME ADJUNCTIVE THERAPIES

As I've mentioned, for treatment of cavitations, the use of Hyperbaric Oxygen Therapy has been recommended in conjunction with surgery. HBOT is the administration of oxygen at high atmospheric pressure. This therapy involves frequent (3 or more times per week), prolonged treatments (usually 30 days for one hour or more each) in a special chamber where oxygen is delivered at increased atmospheric pressure. The protocol recommended by Dr. Hussar for cavitation patients is 90-minute treatments five times per week for 20 sessions at a pressure of 2.4 ATA (atmospheres absolute), with an additional 10 or 20 sessions if needed. According to Dr. Hussar, "It is ideal and usually much better for healing if the patient has at least 4 to 6, or possibly 10 treatments, prior to surgery, followed by 10 or more after." Since HBOT has been used successfully for treatment of gangrene, infections and vascular disorders (as well as a host of other conditions involving insufficient oxygen supply to all parts of the body), it can be a very appropriate therapy for post-surgical treatment of cavitations. Although surgery will remove the bulk of necrotic tissue, HBOT can theoretically deal with any remainder, and also help reverse the ischemic conditions that gave rise to the problem to begin with. I have to say, however, for me, HBOT did not appear to help.

Another therapy which may hold promise for those seriously affected by jawbone cavitations and other oral foci is one that medicine seems to have largely forgotten: Autohemotherapy. This therapy involves injection of one's own blood into the body. Some variations of autohemotherapy involve treating the drawn blood with such substances as ozone or ultraviolet light before returning it to the body. S. Hale Shakman, author of *The Autohemotherapy Reference Manual*, a well-documented review of literature on this obscure subject, suggests that the therapeutic value of such practices may lie as much or more in the autogenous injection as in the treatment of the blood with exogenous substances. Shakman hypothesizes that the blood itself, when injected immediately after removal, acts as an autovaccine, due to the presence of antigens which stimulate antibody production. Various forms of autohemotherapy were used widely from the early 1920s to the early 1940s and had been proven effective against a wide range of disorders, Shakman reveals. This suggests that the simple extraction of a few cc's of blood from a vein and its immediate re-injection into a muscle is perhaps the simplest, safest and most effective form of the therapy. *The Autohemotherapy Reference Manual* is available through the following web site: www.instituteofscience.com.

Shakman has also chronicled the work of the late E. C. Rosenow, MD, which provides important adjunct information on the subject of oral foci. Rosenow, head of the Department of Experimental Bacteriology of the Mayo Clinic from 1915 to 1944, "identified causative organisms for a wide range of diseases — [including] diabetes, epilepsy, multiple sclerosis and schizophrenia – and traced them to their source in oral foci," according to this author. Rosenow also developed special vaccines, made from the patient's own disease organisms, for treating these focal infections. Unfortunately, prominent as this respected researcher was, his work on oral foci, like the research of Dr. Weston Price, seems to have fallen into obscurity. Our very survival may depend upon resurrecting this lost information . . .

In her most recent book, *The Cure for All Advanced Cancers,* Dr. Hulda Clark states that the rare earth elements known as "lanthanides" play a major role in preventing the healing of cavitation sites. These, she maintains, are responsible for local immune loss, as they suppress white cell function. Since these elements have a magnetic quality, Dr. Clark recommends taping an extremely low gauss magnet to the base of the neck to eliminate them from the jawbone. (See her book for details – and follow them exactly) She claims success with this simple procedure.

Bob Jones, the man who gave us the Cavitat machine, has further contributed to our understanding of cavitations by a chance finding he made in 10/98. At that time he observed the presence of a mutated gene (C-677 and L-677) in a majority of people suffering from jawbone cavitations. This particular gene controls homocysteine levels by suppressing the enzyme (methylene tetrahydria folate reductase) that regulates levels of this amino acid. High levels of homocysteine have been positively correlated with greatly increased risk of coronary infarction (heart attack). Jones contends that unstable homocysteine levels will affect the jaw first if there has been trauma (such as tooth extraction, drilling, etc.) to it, creating 'infarctions' there in the form of cavitations. An estimated 65-85% of the population are affected by this genetic mutation, according to Jones.

Here again, the solution eludes us. We do know, however, that high homocysteine levels are a factor in clotting anomalies (tendency to excessive clotting, thick blood) found in a majority of cavitation patients. Therefore, treatment aimed at thinning the blood can theoretically help those suffering from chronic cavitation problems. Aspirin and heparin can accomplish this, but like all drugs, they have undesirable side effects. Jones is partial to the use of COQ10 (a co-enzyme) and garlic. Proteolytic enzymes, such as bromelain, can have the same blood-thinning effect as aspirin, without the adverse side effects.

Additionally, it has been demonstrated that homocysteine levels can be kept in check with supplements of the B vitamins folic acid, B6 and B12. These should be taken in conjunction with a complete B complex source.

One of my readers recently called my attention to the work of Meir Schneider (from the Self Healing Center in San Francisco) involving tension reduction through movement. The movement of a specific body part increases circulation and metabolic activity in that area. In dealing with osteoporosis, Meir employs a bone tapping exercise which may well be applicable to cavitations. The movement and tapping can be combined, as suggested by Meir for my reader, Mitch, following cavitation surgery. The suggested protocol consists of tapping (of the jaw) for about 5 minutes four times a day while simultaneously doing the following: Smiling, puffing cheeks, opening/closing the jaw, moving the jaw from side to side and moving it in circles. Slow, deep breathing and tapping is recommended in conjunction with the execution of these movements.

In an effort to alter the environment which gives rise to cavitations, some experimentation has been done with "Essential Microorganisms" (EMs). EM technology, developed in Japan in 1968, involves the introduction of a variety of helpful, regenerative microorganisms into a weakened terrain in order to strengthen it against the effects of harmful microorganisms. The technology, originally developed for increasing agricultural yield, has also been applied to the terrain of the body. Steven A. Swindler, DDS, of Tuscon, AZ, has pioneered dental applications of EMs. He proposes "irrigation of cavitation sites to eliminate 'seeds' of future NICOs." Such application of EMs is being made experimentally today by a select number of dentists.

The person dealing with chronic jawbone cavitations may, due to the prolonged stress to the body, also be suffering from another widespread but underdiagnosed condition: Wilson's Syndrome. Wilson's Syndrome is a stress-related thyroid disorder involving a functional impairment in the conversion of T4 (the thyroid hormone, thyroxin) to T3 (liothyronine), the active thyroid hormone. Where it is present, body temperature is sub-normal and enzyme function becomes impaired. This makes recovery from cavitations, or any other disorder, difficult. For more information on this important condition and how to effectively treat it, contact the Wilson's Syndrome Foundation at 1-800-621-7006, or check out their website (www.wilsonssyndrome.com).

I have employed some of the adjunct therapies de-scribed in this section. While healing is by no means yet complete, there has been some improvement in my overall condition. I am still in the process of detoxifying my body from the effects of years of hidden infection. Detoxification plays a vital role in recovery from cavitation surgery. And it takes time – and patience. Detoxification is an important foundation upon which to build.

Nutrition is another key element in any recovery plan. Intake of appropriate foods and dietary supplements, as well as avoidance of toxins (in food, water and the environment) can significantly accelerate the healing process.

BOOSTING RECOVERY – THE NUTRITION CONNECTION

Nutrition is a powerful tool in building bodies. Price's epidemiological studies demonstrated not only the efficacy of a natural whole food diet, but also the devastating effects resulting from the introduction of sugar and white flour into the diet.

The reason these products are so destructive is that they have undergone a 'refining' process which strips them of literally dozens of essential nutrients. The trace minerals lost in the refining process are the very nutrients needed for carbohydrate combustion. When we eat a steady diet of refined carbohydrates (sugar and white flour products), our bodies are forced to rob their own storehouses of chromium, manganese, cobalt, copper, zinc and magnesium, the minerals needed to digest these foods. Ultimately, we exhaust our body's storehouses and consequently lose our ability to properly digest carbohydrates. The result is that they ferment or rot (causing us to experience indigestion, gas, bloating), adding to the toxic burden of the body.

Refined carbohydrate consumption also causes sodium leaching (from the stomach, diminishing hydrochloric acid production) and calcium leaching (from bones, interfering with normal skeletal development) to buffer excess acid. By depleting the body of its storehouse of minerals, we deplete our alkaline reserves as well, so that pH (acid/ alkaline) balance cannot be maintained. Since proper pH is critical to mineral assimilation (as well as many other vital functions), the body is then unable to assimilate certain minerals needed to produce enzymes. In the face of enzyme deficiency, digestion is further impaired – and the body's ability to heal is seriously compromised. As our supply of *digestive* enzymes is depleted, the body is forced to recruit its *metabolic* enzymes to perform digestive functions.

These metabolic enzymes are then unavailable to assume their normal function of repairing body tissue. By speeding up chemical reactions within cells, metabolic enzymes normally aid in energy production and detoxification, enabling the body to heal. When needed instead for digestive purposes (a top priority of the body), metabolic enzymes are unavailable to do their normal "damage control" job.

WHOLE, ALKALINE-FORMING AND RAW

As you can see from the above scenario, the habitual consumption of refined foods triggers a cascade of negative events having the net result of greatly reducing the body's healing potential due to mineral and enzyme deficiencies. To reverse this downward spiral, it is necessary to completely eliminate refined foods from the diet, to substitute whole grains for white flour products and to abandon the use of white sugar altogether. If you must have a sweetener, try the herb, stevia, in liquid or powdered form. It has none of the adverse effects of other concentrated sweeteners and, in fact, has actually been demonstrated to help *stabilize* blood sugar levels. And – it won't contribute to tooth decay!

Refined oils must also be eliminated from the diet. Substitute 'unrefined' or 'cold processed' oils, and be sure to include those rich in the essential omega-3 and omega-6 fatty acids. Fish oil is rich in Omega-3s. Flaxseed oil features omega-3, but provides both. It can only be used raw. For cooking, I recommend use of olive oil or unrefined coconut oil (which can withstand very high temperatures without becoming rancid).

To rebuild the body's alkaline reserve, we need to incorporate more fruits and vegetables into the diet. These foods would ideally make up about 75-80% of the diet.

If you are dealing with candidiasis (overgrowth of the fungal form of the candida yeast germ) however, you will need to forego the fruit, as well as a number of other specific foods. Following metal detox, and once candida and other infections (including parasites) have been cleared from the system through diet and special supplements, it is imperative to restore proper pH (slightly *acid*) to the colon and replenish its population of beneficial lactobacteria. A whey supplement, as well as use of probiotics (acidophilus, bifidus, etc.) can be helpful in this regard.

Once colon cleansing has been accomplished, the overworked and possibly malfunctioning liver will also need to be cleansed and rebuilt, and the digestive process normalized. The liver, stomach (together with the duodenum) and colon are organs involved with assimilation/ detoxification, digestion and absorption/elimination respectively. These organs constitute what Dr. Jack Tips describes as "the liver triad" in *Your Liver . . . Your Lifeline.* This book, based on the pioneering research of the late Stuart Wheelwright, gives the details of an excellent program for revitalizing the liver triad. Cleansing of the liver/gall bladder can be accomplished through a special cleansing procedure. Many versions of this cleanse featuring apple juice, olive oil and a few other ingredients, have been used to successfully rid these organs of stones.

To re-build health, you will also want to increase the amount of raw food consumed. Raw foods contain food enzymes which provide enough enzymatic activity to digest them, allowing the body to conserve its own enzymes. Food enzymes are destroyed at temperatures above 116 degrees, so any cooked foods we eat will rob the body of enzymes. Ideally 50% or more of the diet would consist of uncooked foods. The body will become increasingly able to tolerate raw foods as health is restored. Gradually increase the amount you consume. Also, you will want to soak nuts and seeds overnight in water to deactivate enzyme inhibitors, making them more digestible. Grains should also be soaked to improve digestibility.

I highly recommend eating an abundance of organic (or pesticide-free) produce and following the principles of the *Pro Vita! Plan* described in Jack Tips's book of the same name. This plan was devised by Stuart Wheelwright, who had an impressive grasp of the *energetic*, as well as the chemical properties and effects of food. It incorporates many of the above principles in a user-friendly eating plan which is beyond the scope of this book to describe.

ENZYME SUPPLEMENTS

Since the neurotoxic chemicals produced by bacteria in cavitation sites kill many critical enzymes in the body, enzyme supplementation following surgery is of utmost importance. Although the increased intake of raw foods can help conserve the body's enzyme supply, these foods contain only enough enzymes to digest that specific food in which they are contained. There is none left over with which to digest cooked food. Since it is neither practical nor advisable to consume a 100% raw diet in today's world, we are faced then with the problem of how to assist the body with digestion of the cooked foods we eat. The obvious solution is the ingestion of exogenous enzymes. By taking a supplement which contains such important enzymes as protease (to digest protein), amylase (to digest carbohydrates) and lipase (to break down fat) at meal time, we assure proper digestion. We also take considerable stress off the body and increase its resistance, for we are liberating metabolic enzymes which can then do their intended job of healing.

There is another way in which enzymes can be used to help heal the body, one which is relevant to the task of repairing the damage done from cavitations. This enzyme protocol involves the ingestion of protease *on an empty stomach*. When consumed with meals, this enzyme will help digest the protein portion of the meal. When taken on an empty stomach, protease will enter the blood stream where it will break down foreign proteins. It is capable of dissolving nearly *any* protein not incorporated into living tissue. Therefore, this enzyme can assist in the breakdown of parasites, bacteria, virus coatings, fungi, cellular debris, undigested protein (a factor in allergies) and toxins in the blood when taken on an empty stomach. Taken in this manner, it takes a load off the immune system, which can then function more efficiently.

A few days before cavitation surgery, I began taking a large amount of protease between meals; I believe it was 4-6 capsules three times per day. I continued at that high level through the three days of my first surgery, then tapered off to a maintenance dose of 3 capsules twice a day. I also used, and continue to use, digestive enzymes with every meal and snack.

Although I consider enzyme supplementation a *must* in preparation for cavitation surgery and in recovery from it, there is another class of nutrients I believe to be even more important – minerals!

MINERALS

As basic as enzymes are to our health, minerals are actually more important. Acting as coenzymes, they become catalysts, making enzyme functions possible. Not only enzymes, but *all* nutrients require minerals for their activity. All bodily processes depend on the action of minerals.

Mineral deficiency, especially trace mineral deficiency (those minerals needed in small amounts) is widespread today because of mineral depletion of our soils and nutrient-depleting food processing procedures (such as refining). Our foods have become so seriously deficient, that it was found to take 15 ears of corn grown in 1980 to equal the mineral content of one ear grown in 1920.

Senate Document #264 stated the problem this way: "No man of today can eat enough fruits and vegetables to supply his system with the mineral salts he requires for perfect health, because his stomach isn't big enough to hold them." Senate Document #264 was written in *1936!* The situation today with regard to mineral depletion of our soils and food is a critical one, making some form of mineral supplementation essential. It is also very important to remineralize purified or distilled water by adding a liquid mineral supplement to it. One teaspoon of a liquid electrolyte formula containing trace minerals to one gallon of purified water should do the job.

OTHER NUTRIENTS

When it comes to nutrition, I am very whole food oriented and seek to minimize the number of supplements I take. Rather than taking high potency vitamin and mineral supplements, I prefer to incorporate 'super foods,' such as bee pollen, lecithin, rice bran, goat whey, barley grass, wheat grass, spirulina, chlorella and nutritional yeast into my diet. These foods are nutrient dense and present their important nutrients in synergistic combination with other lesser-known nutrients. Such synergy enhances uptake and utilization of nutrients and guards against disruption of balance.

Most of the above mentioned super foods – and many others — are available in a variety of blendable food powders on the market today. These are highly nutritious, but can be over-stimulating to the system if they contain a large number of ingredients. It may therefore be best to start with a single super food, keeping intake moderate.

Despite my preference for whole foods, I acknowledge that it is sometimes appropriate to consume therapeutic levels of specific nutrients for periods of time when the body is under stress (and cavitations and cavitation surgery are *certainly* a big time stress). I do believe, however, that the use of such nutritional supplements should be based largely upon *established* need. There are a number of laboratory tests that analyze blood, urine, saliva, and hair, which can provide information about your nutrient levels. A holistic health care practitioner should be able to help you in this regard. One particularly helpful analysis I've found is a special one that looks at the standard blood profile in a non-standard way to determine a number of factors, including the body's mineral and electrolyte (dissolved mineral salts that carry a charge) status. This unique analysis, which gives valuable information about cell function, is available through Lynne August, M.D., of Health Equations. Check out her website at www.healtheqs.com. The Health Equations' Lyte Solution Concentrate is excellent for remineralizing purified or distilled water.

Following cavitation surgery, you will need appropriate nutritional support to detoxify the body, increase circulation to the jaw, regenerate (and detoxify) the jawbone and enhance immune function. Regardless of the specifics of your individual supplement program, the effects will be noticeably enhanced by the inclusion of minerals, enzymes and super foods. For a more in depth discussion of nutrition, the reader is referred to my latest book, *The Terrain is Everything* (Power of One Publishing).

SOLUTION UNKNOWN

Late in 1999 the new sonogram equipment for detecting cavitations finally became available. The "Cavitat" machine, now being introduced to the medical and dental professions, promises to be a significant diagnostic aid which will make possible substantial progress in the area of cavitation research. For people like myself who have already had cavitation surgery, it will yield important information about progress of the healing and also identify those areas of the jawbone needing further treatment. Hopefully, by allowing the surgeon to visualize the dimensions of a cavitation site, the Cavitat machine will help him/her to thoroughly remove all necrotic material and thus obviate the need for multiple surgeries frequently performed on cavitation patients.

I was introduced to the Cavitat in 1998 at the Second Annual International Congress of Bioenergetic Medicine. Their program guide gave the following description of the device:

> The Cavitat is an acoustic sound-wave diagnostic instrument that provides a 3-D perspective image of the interior of the jawbone at suspected osteomyelitis sites. The Cavitat was designed for the needs of dental surgeons who require a more positive method to identify and accurately locate necrotic lesions, which are far more prevalent than previously suspected. In clinical tests with over 600 patients, the Cavitat performed without a single false positive or negative and has indicated ischemic osteonecrosis in detail. Following the successful detection by the Cavitat, a significant number of patients have undergone surgery to remove these lesions. These patients have begun to recover from long-suffered systemic illnesses.

I was fortunate to have the opportunity to speak at length with the Cavitat's inventor, Bob Jones, at the conference. Bob is an engineer who became completely disabled in 1992 with a speculative diagnosis of ALS, resulting from cavitations. After multiple cavitation surgeries and extensive mercury detoxification, he has almost completely recovered, is fully mobile and quite active.

Bob began work on the Cavitat in the same year in which he became disabled. He launched laboratory trials two years later and clinical trials three years after that. Over the years of developing the Cavitat, Bob has done literally thousands of scans. At the time I first spoke with him in 1997, he had found severe ischemic osteonecrosis and osteomyelitis in every single one of the 4000+ scans he had done on root canal sites. These same lesions were found in 94% of wisdom teeth extraction sites.

The Cavitat results are not difficult to interpret: Necrotic bone shows up in red and yellow, while healthy bone is green. In a scan done at the end of 1999, I was distressed to see a good deal of red, both in edentulous areas which were previously surgerized and in areas of the jaw where restoration-free teeth remain. Apparently the necrosis has spread, affecting the bone underlying "good" teeth. This is a disturbing finding, for which no solution currently exists. I remain encouraged nonetheless by the small improvements I've seen in my overall health.

While I continue the quest for what Dr. Hussar calls my health "Grail," at least now I know what I am dealing with and what I am trying to do. Much of the mystery of my long-standing illness has been taken away, replaced by the knowledge contained in this manuscript. As more information on the subject of cavitations becomes available, the potential for improvement in my prognosis increases.

To find a biological dentist in your area, contact DAMS (1-800-311-6265), the Holistic Dental Association (970-259-1091), the Environmental Dental Association (800-388-8124) or the American Academy of Biological Dentistry (P. O. Box 856, 107 Quien Sabe, Carmel Valley, California 93924). For up-to-date information on cavitation research and treatment, as well as related topics, inquire about the *Cavitations Plus Quarterly* by e-mailing susan@healthcarealternatives.net or contacting Power of One Publishing. As of this writing, *CPQ* is no longer in print, but back issues are available, and publication may resume in the future. Also, check out my website at www.healthcarealternatives.net.

AFTERWORD

Since the publication of the original edition of this book in 1998, I have heard from many readers who have been struggling with cavitation problems and related health issues. Some have reported great benefit from surgery; others have had only limited benefit or temporary relief. The latter have had the procedure repeated, often many times. I don't know what percentage of patients recover fully following cavitation surgery, nor what percentage go on to have the procedure repeated, although this would be important information for practitioners as well as researchers to have. I'd like to know who heals, who doesn't, and why.

Since I have had multiple surgeries and still have jawbone problems, I've sometimes been asked by others why they should even bother to treat their cavitations. This is a perfectly legitimate question. In response, let me say that the outcome of any medical or surgical procedure is never guaranteed. Prognosis is influenced by many variables: age and general health of the patient, severity of his/her problem, duration of the problem, skill of the attending physician, treatment protocol used, etc. Obviously the sooner the problem is addressed, the better the chance of a favorable outcome. To do nothing, on the other hand, guarantees an unfavorable outcome. Prevention is always our best medicine. Early intervention is second best. Without treatment, the condition is sure to get worse. The degree of improvement that can be expected with treatment depends largely on the degree of chronicity.

I remain convinced that surgical treatment of osteomyelitis/osteonecrosis of the jawbone is necessary. However, it appears that surgery is not always *sufficient.* Serious detoxification, both of the body as a whole and of the jawbone in particular, seems to be also in order. The jawbone tends to be a repository for toxins such as chemicals and heavy metals. This environment serves as a breeding ground for all types of microorganisms (including parasites) and their toxic byproducts. Until that environment is changed, the conditions to which it gives rise (cavitations, etc.) will not be eliminated. Detoxifying the jawbone is problematic due to poor blood supply to the area affected by cavitations. Local applications of a healing poultice, held on the jaw area with a facial harness, may be of assistance in this regard.

Although I have heard reports of people benefiting from injections of Sanum remedies into the jawbone, I want to say clearly that this has NOT been my experience. In fact, my experience has led me to believe that this practice can potentially aggravate the problem and cause a spreading of the cavitation(s), as it appeared to have done with me.

It seems to be extremely important for the patient's body to be ready for surgery. A large part of that readiness is making sure the organs of elimination (skin, lungs, colon, kidneys, liver) and the lymphatic system are draining properly, so that toxins have an escape route, a way out of the body, once they are pulled from organs. If elimination is blocked, detoxification efforts will fail, and the patient may feel worse. Also, we do not want to start pulling toxins such as mercury out of the body if the liver and kidneys are too weak to handle the elimination. Heavy metal detox can perhaps most safely be accomplished through the skin in the form of sauna therapy and body soaks.

Another important aspect of detoxification is elimination of all toxic materials in the mouth. This includes all bio-incompatible materials (metallic and non-metallic) and dead teeth. Root canal filled teeth obviously qualify as dead teeth. I've recently learned, however, that dead teeth are not always easy to detect. My own experience with one led me to this realization. The story of that tooth is interesting and worth telling:

The tooth in question is the one that began my dental nightmare five years ago when it was crowned with in-compatible metallic materials. Although those materials were later replaced with "bio-compatible" ones, the tooth was never the same. It did not cause severe or continuous discomfort, but it was never quite right. It would become irritated at the gum margin when I ate fruit or any acidic food. I lived with the problem because none of the many dentists I'd seen over the years could find anything wrong with the tooth.

Last year I learned, through a European publication (*Heavy Metal Bulletin*), of the significant health hazard posed by palladium alloys used in dentistry. I realized with horror that the incompatible material used on the crown placed on my problem tooth so long ago was 40% palladium. Tooth death is just one of many devastating effects of the placement of palladium-containing dental materials in the mouth. Although I had lost all the teeth behind this one (#20), it had somehow managed to survive the trauma of the incompatible palladium-containing crown and subsequent replacement of that crown. I lived with the minor discomfort described above for many years. Following my last cavitation surgery, however, it began to worsen. No problem with the tooth could be found, however, through use of any of the conventional – or unconventional – diagnostic tools. Finally, I took the initiative and scheduled myself for extraction of that tooth. My dentist could find nothing wrong with the tooth initially and was uncomfortable with the prospect of extracting an apparently "vital" tooth. But, he did a final neuro-kinesiology test, and this time - voila! - #20 showed up as a problem. In addition, this problem was shown to be related to weaknesses in the liver, bladder and colon, the very organs that had been giving me problems.

The extraction was done in conjunction with a re-cavitation of an adjacent edentulous area. The extracted tooth *appeared* normal; however, when the pulp chamber was drilled open, the tooth was found to be "dead as a doornail," in my dentist's words.

That dead tooth had remained in my mouth over the course of three previous cavitation surgeries. The unsuspected source of toxicity had been, no doubt, a significant barrier to healing. This experience helps to explain, I believe, why a significant number of people fail to heal completely or permanently following cavitation surgery. Many may have undetected problems with intact teeth, which impede their progress. Soon after extraction of tooth

#20, another hidden dental problem – a leaky crown – was revealed. When it was removed, yet another hidden problem – a cracked tooth – showed up.

Unfortunately, dentistry is greatly limited in its ability to reliably identify problem teeth, especially if they are asymptomatic or only mildly troublesome. Until very recently, it has been equally limited is its ability to pinpoint cavitation sites. The Cavitat will allow us to do this. It will likely force us into a realization of the enormity of the cavitation problem. Check out Bob Jones' website at www.cavitat.com for more information.

Awareness about the cavitation problem is growing. Information on the subject is starting to appear in print and on-line. There are many excellent websites which deal with dental issues. I would recommend visiting Affinity Labeling Technologies' site (www.altcorp.com). It has links to many other related sites.

My current thinking about cavitations is that they can most certainly be avoided if proper extraction protocol is consistently followed. For people like me, with chronic osteitis, it's too late for prevention, and a cure does not currently exist. I still believe a thorough surgical removal of the necrotic tissue is necessary. However, repeated surgeries can be counterproductive. We need to get it right the first time. The Cavitat machine will hopefully make this possible. We also need to uncover and employ effective adjunctive therapies to maximize the effectiveness of the surgical procedure. Trial and error will ultimately tell us what protocols offer the best results.

A solution to dealing with the cavitation epidemic will be forthcoming when awareness of the situation has reached critical proportions and the political and economic barriers to making available the needed research, diagnostics and treatment have been eliminated. Then the long-suppressed truth will resurface for all to see. That process is in motion now.

POSTSCRIPT TO THIRD PRINTING

Exactly one year after having the above-referenced tooth extracted, I had two other mildly troublesome lower ones pulled - again against the advice of my dentist who could find nothing wrong with them through x-ray or muscle testing. Once again, after these tooth were removed from my mouth, their pulp chambers were drilled open and found to be dry. Lack of blood circulation to these teeth had caused them to die, though there was no x-ray nor kinesiological evidence of a problem. Following extraction of these two teeth, my systemic problems improved somewhat for a limited amount of time. Gradually, I started to feel worse, however, and developed additional symptoms. I would later find out why.

These experiences with extractions convinced me that the removal of dead and dying teeth (which often show no overt signs of trouble) could be a key to complete elimination of oral foci. Sometimes, it seems, surgical removal of necrotic bone from edentulous areas is not enough; we must look at the bone beneath remaining teeth, as well. This is best done with bone sonography. For the chronic cavitation patient, saving the tooth at all costs (as dentists are taught to do), is not necessarily the best policy, for the price paid could be loss of health and even loss of life for the patient.

About six months after having the two tooth extractions discussed above, I learned from examination of my panoramic radiograph by Dr. Hussar (who had not previously seen me) that another root tip from an old wisdom tooth extraction had been left in my upper right jaw when the surgery was performed some thirty years before. The previously removed tip was in the lower right jaw. The panorex also gave indication of problems elsewhere in the upper jaw. My previous surgeries had been primarily on the lower jaw which was now looking generally good.

By this time I was working for CAVITAT Medical Technologies, Inc. and beginning to fully appreciate the value of bone sonography. The CAVITAT scan was showing a basically healthy lower jawbone (now with only six teeth in it) and a largely necrotic upper one. These findings made sense, as my overall condition had begun once again to deteriorate, with some new symptoms, which included a chronically clogged right nostril and pain in my upper right arm.

It was pretty clear to me, based on the above findings, that I was in for more surgery. But the question was, "Who do I go to for it?" Since my previous dentists had missed the buried root tip and dead teeth, I wanted to go to someone else. Through the CAVITAT web site I found Dr. Wesley E. Shankland, DDS, MS, PhD, at www.drshankland.com. Dr. Shankland's advanced degrees in anatomy and expertise in facial pain, coupled with his early awareness of 'bone cavities," give him a good grasp of the cavitation problem. As fortune would have it, Dr. Shankland had just purchased a CAVITAT and completed training on it the day before I saw him in 3/01. His scans of me confirmed the presence of widespread necrosis in the upper jaw. Consequently, I made the difficult decision to have all thirteen of my remaining upper teeth removed so that the jawbone beneath could be cleaned out. The surgical, and later the biopsy findings, confirmed the wisdom of the decision. Four of the anterior (middle) upper teeth were fused to the bone, making it difficult to remove them and indicating their lack of vitality due to avascular conditions. I believe the precipitating trauma in the death of these teeth had been the preparation of my two front teeth for porcelain veneers in 1988. These teeth directly affect the genitourinary system, and interestingly, my interstitial cystitis symptoms began right after those teeth were prepped for the veneers. Apparently, the trauma from the high speed drilling killed the pulp of the teeth and created a focal condition which affected my bladder.

During and following surgery with Dr. Shankland, I experienced significant improvement in my overall condition. Some of the improvement even occurred while I was in the dental chair. As he was working to extract the root tip buried deep in my right maxillary sinus, my right nostril cleared entirely, making it much easier to breathe. By the next day, the pain in my right upper arm had diminished greatly, with increased range of motion. Three days later, the breathing problems associated with my "never the same since" injury of 1982 cleared. For the first time since I could remember, I awakened feeling refreshed and breathing freely. These improvements illustrated dramatically the beneficial systemic effects of oral foci removal, and confirmed for me that the jawbone had, indeed, been the source of long-standing and varied conditions throughout the body.

Following my surgery (in fact, it was the evening after), Dr. Shankland met with me to answer some questions. These questions and his answers appear below:

SUSAN: How long have you been involved in treating cavitations?

DR. S.: Since 1985.

SUSAN: What got you started?

DR. S.: While teaching an anatomy course, a periodontist showed me an article by Dr. Ratner on "bone cavities." I then realized I'd been seeing these lesions all along and just didn't recognize them as pathological. With this realization, I started treating them, initially following Ratner's protocol, then evolving my own, based upon sound anatomical principles. I have refined my surgical technique over 16 years of practice.

SUSAN: You specialize in treating facial pain. What percentage of facial pain patients would you say suffer from jawbone cavitations?

DR. S.: About 20% in my practice.

SUSAN: Are these facial pain patients generally helped by cavitation surgery?

DR. S.: More than half, 55-60%, are helped. Of the remaining 40% who undergo a second surgery (same tooth site and/or an adjacent one), about half will experience significant improvement.

SUSAN: How does your surgical technique compare with that of other dentists?

DR. S.: I always make a full flap and reflect the full thickness of the flap - i.e., expose the whole bone. I am radical in my removal of necrotic bone tissue but very cautious about sinuses and nerves. In fact, I have never done any damage to these. Also, I use minimal force when doing extraction of avital teeth. There are others, in contrast, who, rather than doing full flap surgery, go through the socket or make a "window" with either a hand instrument or a burr. I use both, while continually irrigating the site. Also, I use no vasoconstricting anesthetics, as these reduce the blood supply to the area. I use antibiotics when necessary, natural medicines when possible.

SUSAN: What methods do you use to locate cavitations?

DR. S.: Signs and symptoms, bone sonography (CAVITAT scan), x-rays (both panoramic and periapical). I also use confirmation with local anesthetic where pain is present. I may also use applied kinesiology at times, but do not rely upon it soley.

SUSAN: What are the risks vs. benefits of cavitation surgery?

DR. S.: Benefits and potential benefits include eradication of dead bone, restoration of good blood flow, a halting of the progression of the disease. Also, when all oral foci are removed, their distant effects clear. Why this is so is not entirely understood, but it appears to be the case. I have witnessed on numerous occasions the clearing of systemic problems upon removal of an oral focus.

Potential risks include those of any oral surgery: pain, bruising, infection; only partial improvement; no improvement or worsening of the pain; injury or invasion into the maxillary sinus; permanent injury to the inferior alveolar nerve in the lower jaw and tooth loss.

SUSAN: What is your opinion of non-surgical approaches to cavitation treatment?

DR. S.: If it's dead, it has to come out - surgically! This goes for necrotic bone, as well as other tissue such as the periodontal ligament and root tips left behind following extractions.

SUSAN: How can dentists who want to, learn to perform cavitation surgery?

DR. S.: Since there are not any established protocols, and the skill is not taught in dental school, all that can be done at present is to seek out a current practitioner and learn from him or her. I have recently developed and begun offering an extensive 5-day training course approved for continuing education credits.

SUSAN: What kind of adjunctive therapies do you consider useful for the patient before and after surgery?

DR. S.: Nutritional therapy before and after and Anodyne Infrared (LEDs) applied for 20-30 minutes at a time following surgery. This device increases nitric oxide production. Nitric oxide is a key neurotransmitter in healing. Chiropractic is also useful following extended dental work, especially SOT (Sacral-Occipital Technique) to reposition the bones of the skull.

SUSAN: Why do you think it is that many cavitation patients need to undergo repeat surgery or surgeries?

DR. S.: One reason may be lack of proper diagnosis, not identifying all the affected sites or knowing the size and extent of the lesions. Surgery can also fail if the original surgeon did not take care in handling the bone. If the site is not profusely irrigated, the bone will dry out and die. Also, the use of vasoconstrictors will impair blood supply, making the condition worse. Another possibility is failure to recognize and treat an underlying clotting disorder which is present in many cavitation patients. I also believe that use of artificial bone or other foreign matter as an implant in the surgical site can be harmful and may necessitate repeat procedures. Finally, some surgeons just don't get good primary closure - i.e., tight sutures.

SUSAN: How can we reduce or eliminate the need for repeat surgeries?

DR. S. : Avoid all mistakes listed above, plus do not jump into repeat surgeries too quickly.

SUSAN: That's exactly what I did with my own surgeries, #2 and #3. By retreating the edentulous areas and missing the other problems, no improvement resulted and unneeded stress was put on my jaw - very possibly making the condition worse.

SUSAN: How can we prevent cavitations from forming?

DR. S.: We can first of all try to prevent caries. This is largely a dietary matter, though genetics appears to play a role as well. We should make sure that the dentist cleans out the socket properly when extracting a tooth. We can practice good oral hygiene and avoid any unnecessary restorations, including crown, bridges, implants, veneers placed for cosmetic purposes. Large restorations should also be avoided. Avoidance of root canals is important too — I've found all of these to result in necrosis of surrounding bone. Finally, don't take steroids or birth control pills. Cortisone and estrogen can be precipitating factors in the formation of NICO lesions.

Dr. Shankland has made some excellent points. Like me, he has only recently begun to recognize the jawbone (and ultimately the systemic) damage that results from some apparently harmless routine dental procedures. He, like a handful of other dental professionals, is working tirelessly to correct the problem. This awareness will, I feel certain, ultimately revolutionize the practice of dentistry.

APPENDIX A

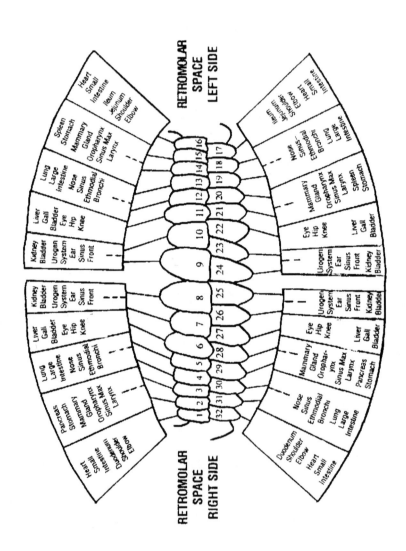

APPENDIX B

Biopsy Reports

From Head & Neck Diagnostics of America
Morgantown, W. Va.

#1 THIS BIOPSY REPORT INDICATES PRESENCE OF BOTH OSTEOMYELITIS AND OSTEONECROSIS IN THE UPPER RIGHT JAW.

BIOPSY REPORT #HN97 - 2219

PATIENT: Susan Stockton
Age: 49   gender: F   Surgery Date: 7/22/97
SOURCE OF SPECIMEN (location):   #1

CLINICAL DIAGNOSIS/DESCRIPTION: NICO type with a possibility of osteomyelitis

GROSS DESCRIPTION OF TISSUE RECEIVED: The specimen consists of numerous tan/maroon, irregular soft tissue fragments measuring 0.7x0.5x0.2 cm in aggregation. The entire specimen is embedded.

MICROSCOPIC DESCRIPTION OF TISSUE: Sections show a thin background film of hemorrhage and fibrin in which are embedded numerous fat globules and apparent oil cysts from fat necrosis. Also embedded are fragments of degenerated collagenic connective tissue with occasional embedded chronic inflammatory cells and with occasional attached bone trabecula which appear viable. A few small fragments of hematopoietic/fatty marrow are present and appear unremarkable. Several small mixed bacterial colonies are noted and presumed to be surface contaminants. Abundant surgical bone dust is seen but none of the bone appears to be necrotic. There is no evidence of malignancy.

MICROSCOPIC DIAGNOSIS: Chronic nonsuppurative osteomyelitis with overtones of osteonecrosis, maxillary right tuberosity.

NOTE: The above diagnosis is based on the interpretation of small tissue fragments and takes into account the cavitation noted at surgery. It is difficult to say which came first, the osteomyelitis or the osteonecrosis, but the inflammatory change seemed to be more dominant.

#2 **THIS BIOPSY REPORT SHOWS OSTEOMYELITIS IN THE UPPER LEFT JAW**.
BIOPSY REPORT #HN97 - 2311

PATIENT: Susan Stockton
Age: 49   gender: F   Surgery Date: 7/22/97

SOURCE OF SPECIMEN (Location): 15-16

CLINICAL DIAGNOSIS/DESCRIPTION: NICO with osteomyelitis and granulation tissue

GROSS DESCRIPTION OF TISSUE RECEIVED: The specimen consists of one white/maroon, cystic/irregular soft tissue mass measuring 0.5x0.4x0.2 cm. The entire specimen is embedded.

MICROSCOPIC DESCRIPTION OF TISSUE: Sections show that this specimen consists predominately of a degenerated and rather avascular collagenic connective tissue containing occasional chronic inflammatory cells and one fragment of bone which appears to be undergoing resorption and appears non-viable. There is no epithelium present and there is no evidence of malignancy.

MICROSCOPIC DIAGNOSIS: Chronic fibrosing osteomyelitis, maxillary left second and third molar areas.

NOTE: The above diagnosis presumes that this tissue is not from the apex of a non-vital tooth. The histology is also consistent with a chronically inflamed periapical scar, which led me years ago to call one of these lesions "residual periapical scar" in an edentulous jaw.

#3 **THIS BIOPSY REPORT INDICATES PRESENCE OF ISCHEMIC OSTEONECROSIS IN THE LOWER LEFT JAW.**

BIOPSY REPORT #HN97 - 2312

PATIENT: Susan Stockton
Age: 49   gender: F   Surgery Date: 7/16/97

SOURCE OF SPECIMEN (location):   #17, 18, 19, 20

CLINICAL DIAGNOSIS/DESCRIPTION: NICO with oil cyst

GROSS DESCRIPTION OF TISSUE RECEIVED: The specimen consists of multiple, cancellous, hemorrhagic, hard bone fragments measuring 1.0x1.0x0.2 cm in aggregation.

MICROSCOPIC DESCRIPTION OF TISSUE: Sections show cortical and trabecular bone which is immature and appears to be newly formed but has almost no residual osteoblastic activity. The background stroma consists of reticular fatty degeneration with occasional chronic inflammatory cells and occasional calcific and proteinaceous necrotic marrow detritus. Osteocytes are seldom missing from the bone. There is no evidence of malignancy.

MICROSCOPIC DIAGNOSIS: Ischemic osteonecrosis (NICO: Type IIc, poor bone healing), left mandibular molar region.

NOTE: The oil cysts noted at surgery are not seen in the specimen. Perhaps they became broken up in transit or were not placed in the biopsy bottle.

#4 **THIS BIOPSY REPORT INDICATES THE PRESENCE OF OSTEOMYELITIS IN THE LOWER RIGHT JAW.**

BIOPSY REPORT #HN97 - 2318

PATIENT: Susan Stockton
Age: 49   gender: F   Surgery Date: 7/16/97

SOURCE OF SPECIMEN (location): #28, 29, 30, 31, 32

CLINICAL DIAGNOSIS/DESCRIPTION: NICO

GROSS DESCRIPTION OF TISSUE RECEIVED: The specimen consists of multiple small irregular and hemorrhagic bony fragments measuring .7x.5x.3 cm in aggregation. The entire specimen is decalcified.

MICROSCOPIC DESCRIPTION OF TISSUE: Sections show fragments of immature bony trabecula with minimal osteoblastic activity and minimal loss of osteocytes. Attached marrow consists of a loose and degenerated fibrous connective tissue with scattered chronic inflammatory cells in small to moderate numbers. A background film of hemorrhage and fibrin contains occasional fat globules but no apparent oil cyst. There is no evidence of malignancy.

MICROSCOPIC DIAGNOSIS: Chronic nonsuppurative osteomyelitis, posterior right mandible.

NOTE: The above diagnosis presumed all of the teeth in the area were vital. Some of the fibrotic and chronically inflamed tissue fragments are also consistent with periapical granuloma.

Note: Biopsy reports from tissue samples taken during the second surgery in May '98 confirmed poor bone healing and continued presence of osteomyelitis.

Toxicology Reports

REPORTS OF IN VITRO SAMPLE TOXICITY
From Affinity Labeling Technologies, Inc.
University of Kentucky
(Assessed by nucleotide photoaffinity labeling of purified enzymes
treated with sample extract).

Level of Toxicity:

0= <5% inhibition, no observable toxicity to these particular enzymes though others may be adversely affected
1= 5-25% inhibition, slightly toxic
2= 26-50% inhibition, mildly toxic
3= 51-75% inhibition, moderately toxic
4= 76-95% inhibition, extremely toxic
5= >95% inhibition, severely toxic

#1 **THIS TOXICOLOGY REPORTS REFLECTS EXTREME TOXICITY PRESENT IN TISSUE SAMPLES TAKEN FROM THE UPPER RIGHT JAW.**

Patient: Susan Stockton
Age: 49   Sample: #1   Date of Analysis: 8/1/97

ENZYME ASSAYED	% INHIBITION	DEGREE OF TOXICITY
Phosphorylase a	91.9	4
Pyruvate Kinase	88.7	4
Phosphoglycerate Kinase	91.4	4
Creatine Kinase	78.0	4
Adenylate Kinase	83.7	4
Average	**86.7**	**4.0**

#2 **THIS TOXICOLOGY REPORT REFLECTS EXTREME TOXICITY PRESENT IN TISSUE SAMPLES TAKEN FROM THE UPPER LEFT JAW.**

Patient: Susan Stockton
Age: 49   Sample: #15-16   Date of Analysis: 8/1/97

ENZYME ASSAYED	% INHIBITION	DEGREE OF TOXICITY
Phosphorylase a	94.2	4
Pyruvate Kinase	88.5	4
Phosphoglycerate Kinase	89.2	4
Creatine Kinase	76.0	4
Adenylate Kinase	80.1	4
Average	**85.6**	**4.0**

#3 **THIS TOXICOLOGY REPORT REFLECTS EXTREME TOXICITY PRESENT IN TISSUE SAMPLES TAKEN FROM THE LOWER LEFT JAW.**

Patient: Susan Stockton
Age: 49   Sample: #17-19   Date of Analysis: 8/1/97

ENZYME ASSAYED	% INHIBITION	DEGREE OF TOXICITY
Phosphorylase a	94.4	4
Pyruvate Kinase	91.3	4
Phosphoglycerate Kinase	90.9	4
Creatine Kinase	70.2	3
Adenylate Kinase	88.5	4
Average	**87.1**	**3.8**

#4 **THIS TOXICOLOGY REPORT REFLECTS EXTREME TOXICITY PRESENT IN TISSUE SAMPLES TAKEN FROM THE LOWER RIGHT JAW.**

Patient: Susan Stockton
Age: 49   Sample: #28-32   Date of Analysis: 8/1/97

ENZYME ASSAYED	% INHIBITION	DEGREE OFTOXICITY
Phosphorylase a	95.7	5
Pyruvate Kinase	92.4	4
Phosphoglycerate Kinase	91.3	4
Creatine Kinase	75.1	4
Adenylate Kinase	88.5	4
Average	**88.4**	**4.2**

Note: An analysis of material from the cavitation at site #16 done after my second surgery in May '98 showed an overall toxicity rating of 71%, a reduction of 15.5% in level of enzyme destruction, showing moderate toxicity.

*BRIEF SYNOPSIS OF THE NORMAL ACTIVITIES OF ENZYMES UNTILIZED BY ALT FOR IN VITRO TOXICITY TESTING AND THE BASIS FOR THEIR SELECTION

I. *Selection of Enzymes*

The primary criteria used for the selection of enzymes for in vitro toxicity testing by ALT are twofold. The first prerequisite is the enzyme must bind nucleotides such as ATP. This allows for the monitoring of the interaction of the enzyme with radioactive photoaffinity analogs of nucleotides like [32p]2N3ATP using the technique of photoaffinity labeling.

Secondly, the nucleotide binding proteins must be very sensitive to a variety of toxic compounds such as heavy metals (mercury, arsenic, etc.) and chemicals (cyanide, hydrogen sulfide etc.) which inhibit their activity by preventing the interaction of the enzyme with their respective nucleotide. Following these criteria we have selected a group of metabolically important enzymes which serve as extremely sensitive indicators of the presence of toxic compounds in biological samples such as extracts from root canal teeth and cavitations.

This approach is similar to the coal miners of old who carried a canary in a cage into the mines with them. In that day and age there were no detectors to tell the miners when oxygen levels were becoming dangerously low or when carbon dioxide or methane gas levels were approaching toxic levels. Instead they relied on the canary which would hopefully show signs of toxicity before they too were overcome. Likewise the toxicity test patch by ALT relies on a combination of sensitive nucleotide binding enzymes which will indicate the presence of a toxic compound or compounds in a sample by a decrease in their ability to interact with their respective nucleotides. Since the photoaffinity probes ALT uses are radioactive, we can detect and quantify this inhibition using the combined biochemical laboratory techniques of sodium dodecyl sulfate polyacrylamide gel electrophoresis (SDS-PAGE), autorad-iography, and radioanalytic detection and quantification.

It turns out that the human body contains many such sensitive nucleotide binding proteins, some of which bind ATP like the 5 we have chosen and others such as tubulin and glutamate dehydrogenase which bind GTP, and still others such as isocitrate dehydrogenase and glyceraldehyde 3-phosphate, dehydrogenase, which bind the nucleotide NAD+ — just to name a few. Each of these enzymes is equally crucial for normal cellular functioning and impairment of any would have dire consequences for the affected cells in the individual.

ALT has chosen a combination of 5 commercially available ATP binding enzymes which meet the aforemen-tioned criteria which can be treated together with a toxic sample extract and afterwards photolabeled all at once in the same test tube with [32P]2N3ATP. While each of these enzymes is sensitive to a variety of toxic compounds, the degree of sensitivity to a given toxin often differs among them. For example, a level of a given toxin such as hydrogen sulfide which completely abolishes [32p]2N3ATP photolabeling of phosphoglycerate kinase only partially inhibits photolabeling of adenylate kinase.

The situation may be reversed for another toxin such as methylmercaptan, which inhibits adenylate kinase much more so than phosphoglycerate kinase. Thus using this combination of 5 enzymes we can detect varying levels of many different toxins in a given sample at one time. This allows us to maximize the amount of data obtained from each analysis while at the same time keeping the cost of our test to a level that is affordable to most patients. However, we ask that you keep in mind that just because a given toxin or toxic extract does not adversely affect the 5 enzymes we have chosen, it does not rule out the possibility that other enzymes would be inhibited by these same toxins.

II. Enzyme Functions
1) Phosphorylase a

Phosphorylase a (Phos a) is the active form of the enzyme phosphorylase; the inactive form being referred to as phosphorylase b. Phosphorylase b is converted to phosphorylase a by the phosphorylase kinase which transfers a phosphate group from ATP to the enzyme by the following reaction.

Phosphorylase b (inactive) + ATP ➡ Phosphorylase a (active) + ADP

Phosphorylase is the controlling enzyme in the breakdown of glycogen to glucose. Glucose is the primary fuel the body uses for the production of adenosine triphosphate or ATP. ATP is the body's source of energy for virtually all cellular processes which include everything from muscle contraction to nerve impulse conduction.

2) Pyruvate kinase

Pyruvate kinase (PK) catalyzes the transfer of the high energy phosphate from phosphoenal pyruvate (PEP) to ADP forming ATP and pyruvate by the following reaction:

Phosphoenolpyruvate + ADP ⬅➡ Pyruvate + ATP

Pyruvate kinase is one of the glycolylic enzymes which functions in the breakdown of glucose to ultimately yield energy in the form of ATP. The three enzymatic pathways involved in this complex process are glycolysis, followed by the tricarboxylic acid (TCA) or citric acid cycle and finally the electron transport chain or oxidative phosphorylation. Pyruvate, which is the end product of glycolysis, can then enter the TCA cycle to begin the second phase in the energy production cycle. In addition to its role in the breakdown of glucose to pyruvate, pyruvate kinase also functions directly in the production of ATP in a process referred to as substrate level phosphorylation (as opposed to oxidative phosphorylation).

3)   Phosphoglycerate kinase
Phosphoglycerate kinase (PGK) catalyzes the conversion of the high energy compound 1,3-bisphosphoglycerate and ADP to 3-phosphoglycerate and ADP by the following reaction:

1, 3-Bisphosphoglyccrate + ADP3-Phosphoglycerate + ATP

Phosphoglycerate kinase is another of the enzymes which functions in the glycolytic pathway involving the conversion of 1 molecule of glucose to 2 molecules of pyruvate which can then enter the TCA cycle. Like pyruvate kinase, phosphoglycerate kinase also functions directly in the substrate level production of ATP.

4)   Creatine kinase (CK) catalyzes the reversible phosphorylation of ADP to ATP from phosphocreatine by the following reaction:

Phosphocreatine + ADP ←→ ATP + Creatine

Tissues which have a high demand for energy in the form of ATP such as the brain and muscle utilize creatine kinase to regenerate ATP. Phosphocreatine is formed during times of low energy demand and when needed this phosphocreatine serves as an energy reservoir from which ATP can be rapidly produced by the activity of creatine kinase.

5)   Adenylate kinase
Adenylate kinase (AK) catalyzes the conversion of 2 molecules of ADP to ATP and AMP by the following reversible reaction:

ADP + ADP ←→ ATP + AMP

ATP is directly produced by the forward reaction and the ADP produced by the reversible reaction can be converted to ATP in glycolysis by pyruvate kinase and phosphoglycerate kinase (substrate level phosphorylation) or in the mitochondrial electron transport chain by the FI-ATPase in oxidative phosphorylation.

As one can readily see, all of these enzymes have one very important thing in common, that being each is involved directly in the production of ATP. The body's ability to produce and maintain ATP levels is absolutely essential for life because every cellular process is driven either directly or indirectly by ATP. Since most of these enzymes are found in virtually every cell in the body, inhibiting the activity of any one of these would certainly prove detrimental to the particular tissue or organ that was affected. However, the effect of inhibiting the activity of any one of these enzymes on the overall health and well being of the patient would depend in large part upon where in the body each of these toxins accumulates.

For example, a toxin or combination of toxins which accumulates primarily in the neurons of the brain and impairs the activity of any or all of these enzymes would produce nervous system pathology. Conversely, a different toxin which accumulates mainly in the myocytes of the cardiac muscle causing enzyme inhibition would impair heart functioning.

In addition, how each individual responds to a given level of toxin or combination of toxins may vary depending on the person's own genetic predispositions, clinical history, age, nutritional status, dental history etc. Therefore, while the photochemical based in vitro toxicity assay performed by ALT can detect if toxins are present in the extract from a particular root canal tooth or cavitation, this assay cannot be used to diagnose or predict the clinical outcome from a particular disease. The results of this in vitro assay do suggest that the presence of these toxins in the body could certainly exacerbate or hasten the progression of any ongoing disease processes.

The information provided above is provided by Affinity Labeling Technologies, Inc., University of Kentucky, A-215B ASTeCC Building, Lexington, KY 40506-0286. It is included with their toxicology test results.

APPENDIX C

PLEASE NOTE: The holes shown in my jawbone in the following photographs were not made by the surgeon: They were uncovered by him and cleaned out. The intent of surgery is to remove necrotic tissue and thereby restore circulation to the area so it can heal.

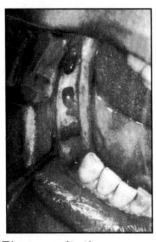

Five cavitations were cleaned out in the lower right jaw, spanning the area of tooth #28 through tooth #32.

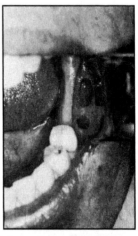

This picture shows 3 cavitations in the lower left jaw. Note that the back 2 are connected, spanning the space between 2nd and 3rd molar sites.

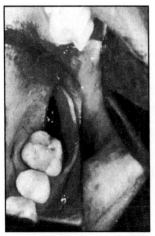

This picture shows another double cavitation, again spanning 2nd and 3rd molar areas; this time upper left jaw. Some visual distortion is present due to the use of a mirror to make the photograph. An additional cavitation was treated in the upper right jawbone, but no photo was taken (after 7 hours in the dental chair, I was too tired to "pose," and the surgeon was ready to go home too!)

NOTES

1. Clark, Hulda Regehr, Ph.D, ND. *The Cure for All Cancers.* ProMotion Publishing, 1993. pg. 47.

2. Huggins, Hal A. *It's All in Your Head.* Avery Publishing Group, 1993. pp. 46-49 and 94).

3. Ibid, pg. 46.

4. Meinig, George E., DDS. "Root Canal Cover Up." *Price-Pottenger Nutrition Foundation Journal,* vol. 18, No. 3, Nov., 1994. pg. 6.

5. Clark, Hulda Regehr. *The Cure for All Diseases.* ProMotion Publishing, 1995. pg. 159.

6. Op. cit., Huggins, pg. 46.

7. Meinig, George E., DDS, FCD. *Root Canal Cover Up.* Bion Publishing, 1993. pg. 183.

8. Op. cit., Huggins, pp. 46-47.

9. Bennett, Peter, ND and Peter Brawn, DDS. "Toxic Teeth." *Townsend Letter for Doctors and Patients,* Aug./Sept., 1997. pg. 146.

10. Levy, Thomas, E., MD, FACC. *Cavitations* video. Peak Energy Performance, 4/19/97.

11. Bouquot, J.E., DDS, MSD. "In Review of NICO, G.V. Black's Forgotten Disease," 1995. pg.1.

12. Ibid.

13. Ibid, pg. 6.

14. Meinig, George E., DDS, FACD. *Root Canal Cover Up.* Bion Publishing, 1993. pg. 193.

15. Tips, Jack, PhD. *Conquer Candida.* Apple-A-Day Press, 1989.

16. "Cavitations and Root Canals...Laura Lee Interview with George Meinig, DDS and Dr. Michael M. LaMarche." *Townsend Letter for Doctors and Patients,* Aug./Sept., 1996.

17. Op. cit., Bennett, pg. 148.

18. Biser, Sam. "Hidden Dental Infections." *The Newsletter of Advanced Natural Therapies,* Vol. 2, No. 5.

19. Meinig, George E, DDS, FACD. *Root Canal Cover Up.* Bion Publishing, 1993. pg. 190.

20. Ibid., pg. 189.

21. Op. cit., Bennett.

22. Meinig, George E., DDS, FACD. *Root Canal Cover Up.* Bion Publishing, 1993. pg. 191.

23. Op. cit., Bouquot, pg. 1.

24. Jerome, Frank, DDS. *Tooth Truth.* ProMotion Publishing, 1995. pg. 280.

25. Op. cit., "Cavitations and Root Canals...", pg. 150.

26. Op. cit., Bouquot, pg. 7.

27. Ibid, pg. 2.

28. Ibid, pg. 3.

29. Ibid., pg. 13.

30. Ibid., pg. 3.

31. Op. cit., "Cavitations and Root Canals..."

32. Op. cit., Bouquot, pg. 13.

33. Biser, Sam. *Health and Healing Newsletter Supplement.* The University of Natural Healing, 4/96. pg. 3.

34. Ibid.

35. Meinig, George E., DDS, FAC. *Root Canal Cover Up.* Bion Publishing, 1993. pg. 184.

36. Op. cit., "Cavitations and Root Canals..."

37. Swilling, Jacob, PhD, ND. "Origin in the Mouth - Where Degenerative Disease Starts." *Health Freedom News,* July/Aug., 1997. pg. 19.

38. Ibid.

39. Biser, Sam. "Hidden Dental Infections." *The Newsletter of Advanced Natural Therapies,* Vol. 2, No. 5. The University of Natural Healing, April, 1996. pg. 6.

40. Ibid.

41. Meinig, George E., DDS. "Root Canal Cover Up." *Price Pottinger Nutrition Foundation Journal,* Vol. 18, No. 3, Nov., 1994. pg. 2.

42. Issels, Josef, Dr. Med.   "More Cures for Cancer." Helfer Publishing, pg. 2.

43. <u>Ibid.</u>

44. <u>Ibid.,</u> pg.3

45. <u>Ibid.,</u> pg. 5.

46. <u>Ibid.,</u> pg.9.

47. <u>Ibid.,</u> pg. 10.

48. <u>Ibid.,</u> pg. 13.

49. <u>Ibid.,</u> pg. 7.

50. <u>Ibid.,</u> pg. 14.

51. <u>Ibid.,</u> pg. 18.

52. Op. cit., Huggins, pg. 52.

BIBLIOGRAPHY

ARTICLES

"Breaking free of Dietary Dogma...An Interview with Sally Fallon." *Spectrum:* #50. Sept./Oct., 1996.

"Cavitations & Root Canals...Laura Lee Interview with George Meinig, DDS and Dr. Michael G. LaMarche." *Townsend Letter for Doctors and Patients.* Aug./Sept, 1996.

Bennett, Peter, ND and Peter Brawn, DDS. "Toxic Teeth." *Townsend Letter for Doctors and Patients.* Aug./Sept., 1997.

Kauppi, Monica. "Slow Recovery in Palladium Exposure." *Heavy Metal Bulletin;* Vol. 5 – Issue 1-2, March, 1999.

Leviton, Richard. "Migraines, Seizures and Mercury Toxicity." *Alternative Medicine Digest,* Issue 21.

Meinig, George, E., DDS. "Root Canal Cover Up." *Price-Pottinger Nutrition Foundation Journal:* Vol. 18, #3. Nov., 1994.

Swilling, Jacob, PhD., ND. "Origin in the Mouth - Where Degenerative Disease Starts. *Health Freedom News.* July/ Aug., 1997.

BOOKS

Clark, Hulda Regehr, Ph.D., ND. *The Cure for All Advanced Cancers.* New Century Press: Chula Vista, CA, 1999.

Clark, Hulda Regehr, Ph.D, ND. *The Cure for All Cancers.* ProMotion Publishing: San Diego, CA, 1993.

Clark, Hulda Regehr, Ph.D., ND. *The Cure for All Diseases.* ProMotion Publishing: San Diego, CA, 1993.

Gates, Donna and Linda Schatz. *The Body Ecology Diet.* B.E.D. Publications: Atlanta, GA, 1996.

Howell, Dr. Edward. *Enzyme Nutrition.* Avery Publishing Group: Wayne, New Jersey, 1985.

Huggins, Hal A., *It's All in Your Head.* Avery Publishing Group: Garden City, New York, 1993.

Jerome, Frank J., DDS. *Tooth Truth.* ProMotion Publishing: San Diego, CA, 1995.

Meinig, George E., DDS, FACD. *Root Canal Cover Up.* Bion Publishing, Ojai, CA, 1993.

Shakman, S. Hale. *The Autohemotherapy Reference Manual.* The Automed Project: Santa Monica, CA. 1998.

Tips, Jack, Ph.D. *Conquer Candida.* Apple-A-Day Press: Austin, TX. 1989.

Tips, Jack, Ph.D. *Your Liver...Your Lifeline.* Apple-A-Day Press: Austin, TX.   1993.

Webster, David. *Achieve Maximum Health.* Hygeia Publishing: Gardieff, CA. 1995.

NEWSLETTERS

Biser, Sam. "Hidden Dental Infections." *The Newsletter of Advanced Natural Therapies,* Vol. 2, No. 5. The University of Natural Healing, Charlottesville, VA.

Heimlich, Jane. "How to Be a Savvy Dental Patient." *Health and Healing Newsletter.* Phillips Publishing, Inc.: Potomac, MD.   April, 1996.

PAPERS

Bouquot, J.E., DDS, MSD. "In Review of NICO, G.V. Black's Forgotten Disease." Edition 4.3, 1995.

Issels, Josef, Dr. Med. "More Cures for Cancer." Helfer Publishing: E. Schwabe, Bad Homburg, Federal Republic of Germany."

VIDEOS

Levy, Thomas, E., MD, FACC. "Cavitations." Peak Energy Performance, Inc.: Colorado Springs, CO, April 19, 1997.

Leber, Douglas C. "Theory on Dental Foci and Disturbance Fields." Lewisville, TX, 1995.

Current Books by Susan Stockton:

Dynamic Healing through NeuroCranial Restructuring - REVISED EDITION

Beyond Amalgam: The Health Hazard Posed by Jawbone Cavitations - REVISED EDITION

The Terrain is Everything: Contextual Factors that Influence Our Health

Health Care Alternatives in the Treatment of Alcoholism & Other Addictions

ADD: It Doesn't Add Up. Drug-Free Alternatives for Hyperactivity & Aggression

Super Nutrition for Men (written in conjunction with Ann Louise Gittleman)

About the Author

Susan Stockton, MA, is a recognized researcher, writer and teacher in the field of natural healing. Since 1988 she has taught *Health Care Alternatives* classes to laymen and health care professionals. Her teaching activities led her to write her first book, *The Book of Health,* in 1990 to use as a text for her classes. Since then she has authored and co-authored numerous books and articles on a variety of health-related topics, including nutrition, sick building syndrome, natural healing principles and practices, the effect of light on health, acupuncture, Attention Deficit Disorder, alcoholism and other addictions, jawbone cavitations and more. Susan holds a master's degree in Rehabilitation Studies and has an extensive background in both counseling and adult education instruction.

NOTES

BOOK ORDER FORM

Name (please print) _____

Street Address or P.O. Box _____

City, State, Zip _____

Phone _____

Discount Schedule		Shipping Charges	
2-4 books	- 10%	up to $25.00	- 4.95
5-10 books	- 15%	$25.01 - $50.00	- 6.95
11-15 books	- 20%	$50.01 - $75.00	- 8.95
16-25 books	- 25%	$75.01 - $100	- 10.95
26-35 books	- 30%	$100.01-$150.00	- 12.95
36-50 books	- 35%	$150.01-$200.00	- 15.95
51+ books	- 40%	$200.01+	- 17.95

Retailers: Call for information
regarding trade discounts

*Florida residents please
add 7% sales tax*

For orders outside US call for information.

Qty.	Book Title	Total

Send payment to:

Power of One Publishing
c/o Renew Life
2076 Sunnydale ~~Drive~~ Blvd .
Clearwater, FL 33765-~~1204~~
1-800-830-4778 X246
susan@healthcarealternatives.net

Subtotal	
Tax if Applicable	
Discount	
Shipping	
TOTAL	